The Essential Oils and Remedies Bible for Everyday Use

5 Books in 1 A Comprehensive Guide to Practical Well-Being, Essence and Alchemy Offers a Trove of Essential Oil Recipes for a Rejuvenated, Toxin-Free Lifestyle

Jenna Jacobsen

Table of Content

Book 1: The Essence of Aromatherapy: An Essential Oils Primer

CHAPTER 1: Introduction to Essential Oils

Delving into the world of essential oils opens the door to a realm where ancient wisdom and modern science converge. These oils, more than mere fragrances, are the distilled essence of nature's profound healing power.

The History and Renaissance of Aromatherapy

Tracing the roots of aromatherapy takes us on a journey back to ancient civilizations, where the intertwining of nature and healing practices began. This enduring practice has transcended time and culture, evolving into a critical component of contemporary wellness.

In ancient Egypt, the first recorded use of aromatic oils laid the foundation for what we now know as aromatherapy. Egyptian medicine was renowned for its sophistication, and aromatic oils played a pivotal role not only in health but also in spiritual practices. These oils, with their ethereal fragrances, were integral to the process of embalming, believed to be a conduit to the divine. Pharaohs were anointed with myrrh and frankincense, carrying these sacred scents into the afterlife.

Moving forward to ancient Greece, we encounter Hippocrates, the iconic physician who championed holistic health. Hippocrates' belief in the healing power of nature, particularly through aromatic compounds, was a beacon of wisdom. The Greeks meticulously documented the properties of essential oils, their work becoming a cornerstone for future explorations in this field.

The Roman Empire furthered this legacy, integrating aromatic oils into daily life through their bathing rituals and massages. Here, aromatherapy began to symbolize luxury and indulgence, transcending its medicinal origins.

During the medieval period, amidst the turmoil of the Dark Ages, monasteries across Europe became the guardians of this knowledge. Monks, deeply attuned to the natural world, continued to distill essential oils, preserving and nurturing this ancient wisdom.

The Renaissance marked a rebirth of aromatherapy, aligning with a broader revival of classical learning. This era saw an amalgamation of scientific exploration and natural healing, with significant advancements in botanical studies and distillation techniques.

The modern chapter of aromatherapy began in the early 20th century, sparked by the work of the French chemist René-Maurice Gattefossé. His accidental discovery of lavender oil's healing properties on a burn led to a renewed scientific interest in essential oils. Gattefossé's work paved the way for a deeper understanding of aromatherapy, blending traditional practices with modern science.

This resurgence in natural therapies, particularly in the late 20th and early 21st centuries, has firmly established aromatherapy in the realm of holistic health. The ongoing exploration into the science of essential oils has unlocked new potentials and applications, merging age-old wisdom with contemporary research.

Today, aromatherapy continues to evolve, shaped by a collective desire to reconnect with nature. In our fast-paced, technology-driven world, it offers a bridge back to the earth's natural rhythms. From ancient embalming rituals to modern organic markets, the evolution of aromatherapy reflects our continuous quest for balance and wellness.

As we look to the future, aromatherapy stands at the forefront of holistic health innovation. Its rich history and evolving practice serve not just as a testament to human ingenuity but as a promise of natural healing and harmony. With each new discovery, aromatherapy continues to illuminate our understanding of health, wellness, and our profound connection with the natural world.

Distillation and Extraction Methods

The heart of aromatherapy lies in its essential oils, the very essence of nature's bounty. These oils, potent and fragrant, are born from a meticulous and fascinating process of extraction and distillation, a dance of science and art that has been refined through the ages.

At its core, the extraction of essential oils is an alchemy of sorts, a transformation of raw botanicals into liquid gold that captures the plant's soul. This journey from plant to oil is both complex and intriguing, involving a delicate interplay of time, temperature, and pressure.

Steam distillation, one of the oldest and most common methods, is akin to a gentle coaxing of the oils from their plant hosts. Imagine a vast field of lavender, its purple blooms a sea under the sun. These fragrant blossoms are harvested and placed in a distillation chamber, where steam permeates through the plant material. As the steam rises, it carries with it the essence of the lavender. In a cooling coil, the steam, now infused with the oil, condenses back into water. The oil, lighter than water, floats to the top, ready to be collected. This method is a testament to the delicate balance of nature – too much heat, and the oil's integrity is compromised; too little, and its soul remains unyielded.

Cold pressing, primarily used for citrus oils like lemon and orange, is a method as vibrant as the fruits themselves. Picture a ripe orange, its skin bursting with zest and aroma. In cold pressing, the rind of these fruits is mechanically pressed, bursting the tiny oil sacs within. The resulting liquid, a mixture of oil and fruit juice, is then centrifuged to separate the oil. This method retains the bright, zesty essence of the fruit, unaltered by the heat used in distillation.

Solvent extraction offers a route to capture the delicate fragrances of flowers like jasmine and rose, whose essence can't withstand the rigors of distillation. In this method, the plant material is bathed in a solvent, usually hexane, which dissolves the aromatic compounds. The solution is then filtered and gently heated, leaving behind a waxy substance known as a concrete. Further processing with alcohol yields an absolute – the pure, potent essence of the flower. This method, though complex, unlocks aromas that would otherwise remain imprisoned in the petals.

CO2 extraction, a modern marvel, harnesses the unique properties of carbon dioxide when subjected to high pressure. Under these conditions, CO2 acts as a solvent, pulling out the oil from the plant. Upon release of the pressure, CO2 returns to its gaseous state, leaving behind the pure oil. This method is lauded for its ability to extract oils without using high temperatures, maintaining the integrity and full spectrum of the plant's components.

Each of these methods – steam distillation, cold pressing, solvent extraction, and CO2 extraction – has its own symphony of intricacies, a dance of elements choreographed to extract nature's elixirs. The choice of method is a critical decision, influenced by the nature of the botanicals and the desired characteristics of the final oil.

The journey from plant to oil is not just a scientific process but a form of art. It requires a deep understanding of the plants, an intuition for their secrets and a respect for their fragility. The distiller, much like an artist, must balance the science of temperature and pressure with the intuition of timing and observation.

As we delve into this world of extraction and distillation, we uncover more than just the methods; we discover a narrative of human ingenuity and nature's generosity. These methods are not mere procedures; they are the rites through which the essence of nature is honored and captured.

In this exploration, we come to appreciate the complexity behind each drop of essential oil. The journey of a single drop is a narrative of transformation, a testament to the harmony between human endeavor and nature's gifts. It is a journey that begins in the soil and ends in the soul, a journey where science meets spirit.

As we hold a bottle of essential oil, we are not just holding a product; we are holding the end of a profound journey. This journey of distillation and extraction is a story of transformation, a story that underpins the very essence of aromatherapy. It is a story that celebrates the beauty of nature, the wisdom of tradition, and the innovation of science – a story that is as enriching as the oils themselves.

Understanding Purity and Quality

The essence of essential oils lies not just in their enchanting aromas or therapeutic benefits, but fundamentally in their purity and quality. This crucial aspect is the cornerstone upon which the efficacy and safety of aromatherapy rests. Understanding purity and quality in essential oils is akin to unraveling a complex, intricate tapestry woven from the threads of botanical integrity, extraction finesse, and meticulous testing.

Purity in essential oils is the unadulterated essence of the plant, untouched by synthetic additives or chemical enhancers. It is the pure, unblemished soul of the plant captured in a bottle. However, the path to achieving this purity is fraught with challenges, ranging from agricultural practices to the final stages of bottling.

The journey of an essential oil begins in the very soil where its source plant thrives. The quality of this soil, the air that whispers above it, and the water that quenches its thirst, all play pivotal roles. Organic farming practices, free from pesticides and chemical fertilizers, lay the foundation for pure, high-quality essential oils. These practices ensure that the plants grow in their natural state, unburdened by artificial interventions, thus preserving their innate essence.

Once harvested, the method of extraction becomes the next guardian of purity. Traditional methods like steam distillation or cold pressing, when executed with precision, maintain the integrity of the oil. Modern methods like CO_2 extraction, while more efficient, require a profound understanding of temperature and pressure to ensure that the oil's chemical profile remains unaltered. Each drop of oil is a delicate balance of nature's design and human craftsmanship.

However, the true measure of an oil's purity and quality is revealed in the laboratory. Rigorous testing methods like Gas Chromatography and Mass Spectrometry (GC-MS) are employed to unveil the oil's chemical blueprint. These tests decipher the complex symphony of compounds within each oil, ensuring that no unwanted notes disrupt the harmony. Purity is confirmed when the oil's composition aligns with its botanical identity, untainted by fillers or synthetic imposters.

Beyond chemical analysis, organoleptic testing – a sensory evaluation by skilled aromatherapists – plays a crucial role. This evaluation involves a symphony of senses: the eyes observe the oil's clarity and color, the nose detects its aroma, and the touch assesses its texture. This human element adds a layer of depth to the understanding of an oil's quality, capturing nuances that machines might overlook.

Quality, however, is not just a matter of purity. It extends to the ethical sourcing of plant materials, ensuring sustainability and fair trade practices. It's about respecting the earth and the hands that toil it, ensuring that each bottle of essential oil carries within it a story of ethical stewardship.

Furthermore, quality is also about consistency. A reputable essential oil should maintain a consistent profile batch after batch, a testament to the producer's commitment to standards and excellence. This consistency builds trust and reliability, ensuring that therapists and users can depend on the oil's therapeutic properties.

In an industry where adulteration and misleading claims are not uncommon, understanding and ensuring purity and quality become acts of responsibility. It's about protecting the legacy of aromatherapy, preserving the trust placed in these ancient remedies by those who seek healing and comfort in their embrace.

As we delve into the realm of essential oils, we embark on a quest for truth – a truth that lies in the purity of the oil and the integrity of its source. This quest is a commitment to honoring the bond between humanity and the plant kingdom, a pledge to uphold the sanctity of nature's gifts.

In essence, the purity and quality of essential oils are not mere technical terms but are the heartbeats of aromatherapy. They are the pillars that uphold the practice, ensuring that each encounter with these oils is as authentic and beneficial as nature intended. As guardians of this ancient art, it is our duty to ensure that these pillars remain unshaken, preserving the purity and quality of essential oils for generations to come.

CHAPTER 2: The Fundamentals of Aromatherapy

Embarking upon the exploration of aromatherapy's fundamentals, we invite readers into a realm where the essences of nature are transformed into conduits of healing and harmony.

Essential Oil Profiles: Characteristics and Benefits

Embarking on the journey into the fundamentals of aromatherapy, one must first acquaint themselves with the heart of this practice – essential oils. Each oil, a unique blend of nature's whispers and secrets, holds characteristics and benefits that beckon for a deeper understanding.

Lavender, often referred to as the 'mother of essential oils,' embodies versatility and gentleness. Lavender's floral, herbaceous aroma is more than just a pleasant scent; it's a balm for the restless mind and a haven for troubled sleep. Its compounds, primarily linalool and linalyl acetate, have been studied for their calming effects, making it a staple in stress relief and sleep-promoting blends.

Peppermint, with its invigorating and cooling sensation, is like a breath of fresh mountain air. Its primary component, menthol, imparts a refreshing quality, making it a favorite in alleviating fatigue and enhancing mental clarity. Beyond its uplifting aroma, peppermint has been revered for aiding digestion and easing headaches.

Eucalyptus, a symbol of cleansing and rejuvenation, offers a camphoraceous, crisp scent that seems to open airways and clear minds. Its main constituent, 1,8-cineole, is renowned for its respiratory benefits, making eucalyptus oil a common ally in combating seasonal ailments and improving respiratory health.

Lemon, the epitome of brightness and clarity, brings a zesty, uplifting aroma to the blend. Rich in limonene, lemon oil is celebrated not just for its refreshing scent but also for its cleansing properties. It's often utilized in purifying air, enhancing mood, and even in skin care for its ability to brighten and tone.

Tea tree oil, with its robust, medicinal aroma, stands as a powerful warrior against impurities. Primarily composed of terpinen-4-ol, it's highly regarded for its purifying qualities. Tea tree oil is a common choice for topical applications, particularly in skin care, where it battles blemishes and promotes clarity.

Rosemary, redolent of the Mediterranean breeze and herbal gardens, offers more than just culinary delight. Its main components, such as 1,8-cineole and camphor, lend it properties that invigorate the mind and body. Rosemary is often turned to for its ability to enhance memory, support circulation, and invigorate the senses.

Frankincense, often dubbed the 'king of oils,' carries an ancient mystique in its warm, balsamic aroma. Comprised of compounds like alpha-pinene and limonene, it's revered for its ability to soothe the mind and rejuvenate the skin. Its grounding aroma makes it a favorite for meditation and spiritual practices.

Ylang Ylang, with its rich, floral scent, is like a walk through a tropical garden. Its main constituents, including germacrene and caryophyllene, contribute to its reputation as an oil that soothes the heart and mind. Ylang Ylang is often employed in blends for stress relief and is also celebrated for its beautifying properties in skin and hair care.

Each essential oil, a complex character with its own story, offers a spectrum of therapeutic benefits. Understanding these profiles is like learning a new language – the language of nature. It enables us to listen to the subtle cues of our bodies and the environment, responding with the appropriate aromatic symphony.

This understanding also guides us in creating blends that not just smell divine but also work synergistically for desired effects. Whether seeking relaxation, invigoration, purification, or healing, the knowledge of these oil profiles equips us to harness their benefits effectively.

The characteristics and benefits of essential oils are akin to a kaleidoscope of nature's healing powers. Each turn, each blend, reveals a new pattern, a new potential for health and well-being. As we delve deeper into the world of aromatherapy, this knowledge becomes our compass, guiding us to use these precious oils with respect, understanding, and a sense of wonder.

In exploring these oil profiles, we are not just uncovering the therapeutic properties of each oil; we are also embracing a holistic approach to health. One that respects the wisdom of the past, acknowledges the science of the present, and looks forward to a future where wellness is harmoniously balanced with nature.

Carrier Oils and Blending Basics

In the art of aromatherapy, essential oils are akin to precious gems – potent, concentrated, and powerful. Yet, just as gems require a perfect setting to be worn comfortably and safely, essential oils rely on carrier oils for their effective and safe application. The blending of essential oils with carrier oils is an art in itself, a harmonious balance that enhances the therapeutic properties of the oils while ensuring their safe use.

Carrier oils, often unsung heroes in the world of aromatherapy, are derived from the fatty portions of plants, typically the seeds, kernels, or nuts. These oils are named 'carrier' because they carry the essential oil onto the skin, diluting their intensity and allowing for a gentler experience. Unlike essential oils, which are volatile and evaporate quickly, carrier oils are stable, grounding the essential oils and prolonging their therapeutic effects.

Jojoba oil, a liquid wax rather than a true oil, mirrors the natural sebum of the skin, making it an excellent choice for facial blends. Its stability and resemblance to skin's natural oils allow it to balance oil production, making it suitable for a wide range of skin types.

Sweet almond oil, rich in vitamins E and K, is a nourishing choice for the skin. Its mild, nutty aroma makes it a versatile carrier, blending well with a multitude of essential oils. Ideal for massage, it glides smoothly over the skin, carrying the benefits of the essential oils deep into the tissues.

Coconut oil, with its rich, fatty acid profile, offers a luxurious feel on the skin. In its fractionated form, it remains liquid at room temperature, making it an excellent carrier for topical applications. Its light texture and moisturizing properties make it a favorite for full-body applications.

Grapeseed oil, light and thin in consistency, is a go-to carrier for those who prefer a non-greasy feel. Rich in linoleic acid, it's known for its skin-nourishing properties and is particularly suited for oily or acne-prone skin.

Avocado oil, thick and deeply penetrating, is a treasure trove of vitamins A, D, and E. Its rich, nourishing profile makes it ideal for dry or aging skin, offering deep moisturization and supporting skin's natural barrier.

The art of blending is not just about mixing an essential oil with a carrier; it's about understanding the synergy between different oils. A well-crafted blend considers the therapeutic properties of both the essential and carrier oils, creating a concoction that is greater than the sum of its parts.

When creating a blend, start by identifying the purpose of the blend – be it for relaxation, invigoration, skin care, or muscle relief. This purpose guides the choice of essential oils and the selection of the carrier oil that best complements these properties.

The process of blending requires a gentle touch and a mindful approach. Begin by adding the essential oils drop by drop into the carrier oil, swirling gently to mix. This slow addition allows for the essential oils to integrate fully with the carrier, ensuring an even distribution.

Labeling the blend with its contents and the date of blending helps in tracking its usage and shelf life. Most blends, depending on the carrier oil's shelf life, can be used for several months if stored in a cool, dark place.

In blending, one also learns to appreciate the individuality of each oil – how some essential oils, like lavender, are versatile and blend well with almost any carrier, while others, like eucalyptus, may need a lighter carrier to balance their intensity.

The practice of blending is a journey of discovery – each blend a unique story, each application an experience. It's a dance of scents and textures, a weaving of the therapeutic tapestry that is aromatherapy. As one delves deeper into this art, each bottle of carrier oil and each vial of essential oil becomes a chapter of knowledge, a step closer to mastering the art of healing through nature's bounty.

In embracing the art of blending, we not only harness the power of essential oils but also pay homage to the carriers that bring them to life. It is a practice that calls for respect, understanding, and creativity – qualities that make the journey of aromatherapy an endlessly rewarding one.

Safety Guidelines and Dilution Ratios

Navigating the world of aromatherapy requires not just an appreciation of the oils' fragrances and benefits but also an understanding of their safe and effective use. The essence of safety in aromatherapy lies in respecting the potency of essential oils and recognizing the delicate balance necessary for their optimal use. This understanding is pivotal to harnessing their benefits while ensuring the well-being of those who seek their healing touch.

The first rule of safety in aromatherapy is acknowledging the potency of essential oils. These concentrated plant extracts are far more powerful than their botanical sources. A single drop of essential oil can be equivalent to multiple cups of herbal tea from the same plant. This concentration is not just a measure of strength but a reminder of the need for respectful, judicious use.

Understanding dilution is crucial in the safe application of essential oils. Dilution involves blending essential oils with carrier oils to mitigate the intensity of the essential oils, making them safe for topical application. This practice is not just about reducing the risk of skin irritation or sensitization; it's about maintaining the therapeutic integrity of the essential oils. Proper dilution enhances absorption through the skin and prevents the evaporation of the volatile components of the essential oils.

The guidelines for dilution are not arbitrary but are grounded in research and practice. A general rule for topical application is a dilution ratio of 1-3% essential oil to carrier oil. This ratio provides an effective concentration for most adult users. For children and sensitive individuals, a more conservative approach is recommended, typically a dilution of 0.5-1%.

In specific therapeutic contexts, higher dilutions may be warranted. However, such cases require the guidance of experienced practitioners who understand the nuances of essential oil interactions and the individual's health background.

Besides dilution, the choice of application method plays a significant role in safety. Essential oils can be used in various ways - topical application, inhalation, or diffusion. Each method has its considerations. Topical application requires strict adherence to dilution guidelines, while inhalation should be approached with caution, particularly for those with respiratory issues. Diffusion, while generally safe, should be done in well-ventilated areas and in moderation to prevent overexposure.

Certain essential oils carry specific safety concerns. For instance, oils like wintergreen and bitter almond contain components that can be toxic if used improperly. Citrus oils, beloved for their uplifting scents, are phototoxic and can cause skin reactions if exposed to sunlight after application. Pregnant women, children, and individuals with certain health conditions should exercise additional caution, as some oils can have contraindications.

Labeling and storing essential oils correctly is another aspect of safe practice. Proper labeling ensures correct identification and prevents misuse, while storing oils away from light and heat preserves their integrity and longevity.

Understanding the signs of adverse reactions and knowing how to respond is also key. Skin irritation, headaches, or nausea can be signs of overexposure or sensitivity. In such cases, discontinuing use and seeking advice from a qualified professional is crucial.

Safety in aromatherapy extends beyond individual use. It encompasses ethical sourcing and environmental stewardship. Using sustainably sourced and ethically produced oils not only supports the wellbeing of the planet but also ensures that the oils are of the highest quality, free from adulterants that can compromise safety.

In essence, safety in aromatherapy is about harmonizing our respect for the oils with our understanding of their nature. It's about creating a space where the healing power of essential oils can be embraced fully and safely. This balance of knowledge and respect transforms aromatherapy from a mere practice into a mindful journey of wellness.

As we continue to explore the depths of aromatherapy, let this understanding of safety be our guiding star. Let it illuminate our path as we navigate the rich landscape of essential oils, ensuring that our journey is not only fragrant and therapeutic but also safe and nurturing. In this way, we honor the true spirit of aromatherapy – a practice that is as nurturing as it is healing, as responsible as it is transformative.

CHAPTER 3: Sensory Essentials

Delving into the world of sensory essentials, we embark on an enlightening journey through the realm of aromatherapy, where scents are more than mere fragrances; they are the keys to unlocking profound emotional and psychological responses.

Olfactory System and Emotional Well-being

The journey into the realm of aromatherapy is incomplete without understanding the profound connection between our olfactory system and emotional well-being. This intricate relationship, a dance of scents and emotions, is at the heart of why aromatherapy is more than just pleasant aromas—it's a gateway to emotional balance and mental tranquility.

Our olfactory system, a sentinel at the gates of our brain, is directly wired to the limbic system, the emotional center of the brain. This direct connection is unique in the sensory world, making the sense of smell an immediate, unfiltered pathway to our emotions and memories. When we inhale an essential oil, its molecules travel through the nasal passages to the olfactory receptors, initiating a cascade of neural responses. These responses trigger the limbic system, influencing our emotions, mood, and even behaviors.

Consider the experience of inhaling lavender. Its molecules, upon reaching the olfactory receptors, send signals that stimulate the brain to release calming neurotransmitters. This cascade leads to a sense of relaxation and may even reduce anxiety levels. On the other hand, the zesty aroma of citrus oils like lemon or bergamot can uplift the spirit, promoting feelings of joy and invigoration.

This profound connection has roots in the evolutionary history of humans. The sense of smell was crucial for our ancestors' survival, aiding in the detection of food, predators, and mates. Over time, this sense developed an intimate link with the emotional brain, making it a powerful tool for influencing mood and well-being.

The impact of aromas on emotional health is not just anecdotal; it's backed by scientific studies. Research has shown that certain essential oils can significantly impact mood disorders, stress, and anxiety. For example, a study on orange oil demonstrated its ability to reduce anxiety in dental patients, while rose oil has been found to improve the mood of postpartum women.

But the relationship between scent and emotion is deeply personal. Each individual may respond differently to the same aroma, a testament to our unique emotional landscapes and life experiences. For some, the scent of rose might evoke feelings of love and warmth, perhaps a reminder of a cherished memory. For others, it might bring a sense of comfort, reminiscent of a nurturing presence in their lives.

This individual response to scent is why personalized aromatherapy is so powerful. It allows us to select oils that resonate with our emotional needs and preferences. By understanding our emotional responses to different scents, we can create personalized blends that cater to our specific emotional states—be it to calm, uplift, energize, or comfort.

Beyond personal well-being, the olfactory-emotional connection has broader implications. It's used in various settings, from spas to healthcare environments, to foster an atmosphere of comfort and peace. In hospice care, for instance, aromatherapy is often used to provide emotional solace and reduce anxiety in patients and their families.

In exploring the link between the olfactory system and emotional well-being, we uncover the essence of aromatherapy's power. It's a reminder that our sense of smell is a direct line to the heart of our emotional world. This understanding empowers us to use aromatherapy not just as a way to enjoy pleasant scents, but as a tool to navigate the complex terrain of our emotions.

Creating Personalized Scent Profiles

In the enchanting realm of aromatherapy, the creation of a personalized scent profile is not just an exercise in fragrance selection; it is a journey into self-discovery and sensory harmony. This process is as unique as the individual, reflecting personal stories, memories, and emotions, all interwoven with the subtle language of scents. Crafting a personalized scent profile is akin to painting a portrait, where each aroma adds a stroke of color and texture to the canvas of one's sensory identity.

To embark on this journey, one must first become attuned to the subtle nuances of different essential oils. It begins with exploration and experimentation, where the individual is invited to experience a variety of scents, noting their immediate emotional and physical responses. This sensory exploration is not merely about preference, but about resonance – finding those scents that echo one's inner landscape and emotional needs.

Consider lavender, with its soft, floral notes that often evoke a sense of calm and tranquility. For someone seeking relaxation or a soothing balm for stress, lavender may be a central note in their scent profile. Contrast this with the invigorating freshness of peppermint, which might resonate more with someone who seeks rejuvenation and mental clarity. The scent profile for each individual is a mosaic of such choices, each oil contributing its unique emotional and aromatic signature.

Beyond the individual response, understanding the properties of essential oils is crucial in creating a balanced and harmonious profile. Some scents, like the earthy richness of patchouli or the sweet warmth of vanilla, serve as base notes, providing depth and longevity to the profile. Middle notes, such as the floral elegance of rose or the spicy allure of cardamom, offer body and roundness. The top notes, like the zesty brightness of citrus oils, add a burst of initial freshness, greeting the senses upon first inhalation.

The artistry in crafting a scent profile lies in the blending of these notes, achieving a synergy where each oil enhances the others, creating a harmonious whole greater than its parts. This blending is not bound by strict formulas but guided by intuition and personal preference, allowing the individual's personality and emotional needs to guide the composition.

In creating a personalized scent profile, one must also consider the context in which the fragrances will be used. A profile designed for personal well-being might differ from one intended for a specific environment, like a home or workspace. The former might focus on deeply personal resonances, while the latter might aim to create a welcoming, inclusive atmosphere.

Another dimension to consider is the evolution of scents over time. Just as individuals grow and change, so too might their scent preferences. Thus, a personalized scent profile is not a static entity but a living, evolving expression of the individual. Regular revisiting and tweaking of the profile ensure that it continues to align with the individual's journey and current state of being.

In crafting these personalized scent profiles, we tap into the ancient wisdom of aromatherapy, intertwining it with modern understanding of emotional well-being. This practice transcends the mere act of smelling; it becomes a form of self-expression and emotional nourishment. Each inhalation of these personalized scents serves as a reminder of one's unique journey, offering comfort, motivation, or peace as needed.

Creating a personalized scent profile is thus an intimate dance with the senses, a celebration of individuality, and a testament to the transformative power of aromas. It is an act of self-care and expression, where the mystical world of scents meets the personal narrative, crafting a fragrant story that is as unique as the individual themselves.

The Art of Natural Perfumery

Natural perfumery, a sublime craft that intertwines the essence of nature with human creativity, is an art as ancient as civilization itself. This art is not merely about creating pleasing aromas; it's a profound expression of nature's diversity and complexity, conveyed through the language of scent. In natural perfumery, the perfumer is both an artist and a chemist, blending essential oils, absolutes, and botanical extracts to create a symphony of fragrances that resonates with the soul.

At the heart of natural perfumery lies the understanding of the unique characteristics of each botanical ingredient. These natural essences, each with their own story, are carefully selected and combined to create a fragrance that is not only captivating but also harmonious and balanced. The process begins with a vision, an inspiration drawn from nature, emotion, or experience. This vision guides the perfumer in choosing the right combination of top, middle, and base notes.

Top notes are the initial impression of the perfume, the scents that greet the senses upon the first encounter. Citrus oils like bergamot and lemon, with their fresh and uplifting aromas, are often used as top notes. They are the fleeting whispers of the fragrance, setting the stage for the deeper notes to unfold.

Middle notes, or heart notes, form the core of the perfume. They emerge just as the top notes begin to dissipate. Floral essences like rose, jasmine, and lavender are classic middle notes, lending a soft, rounded richness to the fragrance. They are the storytellers, weaving the narrative of the perfume.

Base notes are the foundation upon which the perfume rests. They linger long after the top and middle notes have faded, providing depth and solidity to the fragrance. Resins such as frankincense, myrrh, and woods like sandalwood and cedarwood are common base notes. They are the memory of the perfume, anchoring the fragrance with their enduring presence.

The art of blending these notes is a delicate balance, requiring patience, skill, and intuition. The perfumer must understand how each essence interacts with others and how they evolve over time. The process is iterative, a series of adjustments and refinements, as the perfumer strives to achieve the perfect harmony between the different elements.

In natural perfumery, the ingredients are more than just scents; they are imbued with therapeutic properties that can affect mood and well-being. Thus, creating a natural perfume is not only an artistic endeavor but also a holistic one. The perfumer must consider not only the aesthetic qualities of the fragrance but also its potential effects on the mind and body.

Sustainability and ethical sourcing are also integral to natural perfumery. With the growing awareness of environmental issues, natural perfumers are committed to using ingredients that are not only pure but also responsibly harvested. This commitment ensures that the art of perfumery contributes positively to the environment and supports the communities involved in the cultivation and extraction of botanicals.

The finished product, a natural perfume, is a reflection of the perfumer's artistry, the essence of nature, and the intangible qualities that make each fragrance unique. It's a personal signature, an invisible accessory that complements the wearer's personality and style.

Natural perfumery is thus a dance with the senses, a celebration of the gifts of nature, and a testament to human creativity. It's an art form that respects tradition while embracing innovation, creating fragrances that are timeless yet contemporary. As we delve into this world, we discover that each bottle of natural perfume is not just a fragrance but a story, a piece of art, a sensory journey that delights and inspires.

CHAPTER 4: Essential Oils in Daily Life

Exploring the realm of essential oils in daily life unveils a world where every drop of these natural elixirs contributes to a harmonious and healthful existence. This chapter delves into the practical and transformative ways essential oils can be woven into the fabric of our everyday routines.

Integrating Aromatherapy into Your Routine

The incorporation of aromatherapy into daily life is a journey towards harmonizing our external environment with our internal state, creating a sanctuary where mind, body, and spirit align. This integration is not about overhauling routines but weaving the subtle yet profound benefits of essential oils into the fabric of our everyday lives.

Morning rituals set the tone for the day. Imagine starting your day with the invigorating aroma of peppermint or citrus oils diffusing through the air, awakening your senses and clearing your mind for the day ahead. These scents, with their uplifting properties, can be a natural substitute for your morning caffeine boost, offering an energizing start without any jitters.

Throughout the day, aromatherapy can be a constant companion, subtly enhancing moments and moods. For the midday slump when focus wanes, a blend of rosemary and lemon can be revitalizing. Just a few drops in a diffuser or on a cotton ball near your workspace can help in regaining concentration and clarity. These oils, known for their ability to enhance cognitive function, can be a gentle nudge to keep productivity and motivation high.

The transition from day to evening is another opportunity to incorporate aromatherapy. As the day's pace slows, the calming scents of lavender or chamomile can be introduced to signal the body and mind to relax. Creating a ritual around this transition, perhaps with a few minutes of inhaling these soothing scents deeply, can be a powerful way to release the stresses of the day and prepare for a restful evening.

Incorporating essential oils into personal care routines also offers a daily touch of luxury and well-being. Adding a few drops of skin-friendly oils like frankincense or geranium to your moisturizer not only benefits the skin but also provides a sensory experience that is both grounding and nurturing. These moments of self-care become more than just routine; they become a ritual of self-love and wellness.

Mealtime can also benefit from the subtle use of aromatherapy. While essential oils should never be ingested without professional guidance, diffusing gentle, appetite-enhancing scents like sweet orange or ginger in the dining area can create a pleasant atmosphere for enjoying meals. It's about creating an environment that complements the food and enriches the dining experience.

The power of aromatherapy extends even to the end of the day, preparing the body and mind for sleep. Creating a bedtime routine with oils like vetiver, known for its grounding properties, or a calming blend of lavender and ylang-ylang can signal to the body that it is time to wind down. This routine could involve a few drops in a bedside diffuser or a soothing massage with these oils diluted in a carrier oil.

The beauty of integrating aromatherapy into daily life lies in its flexibility and personalization. Each person's routine and choice of oils can be tailored to their specific needs and preferences. It's about listening to one's body and mind and responding with the appropriate aromatic therapy.

Moreover, integrating aromatherapy into daily life is about cultivating mindfulness and presence. It encourages a moment-to-moment awareness of our surroundings and our inner state, allowing the subtle power of scents to bring us back to the present.

In essence, integrating aromatherapy into daily routines is about creating small oases of well-being throughout the day. It's a practice that doesn't demand much time or effort but offers significant returns in terms of emotional balance, mental clarity, and overall well-being. As we navigate the complexities of modern life, these moments of aromatic mindfulness can be a source of strength and serenity, a gentle reminder of the beauty and power of nature's essences.

Essential oils for sleep, concentration and energy

Dreamy Lavender Sleep Blend

P.T.: 5 minutes

Ingr.: 10 drops Lavender Essential Oil (Lavandula angustifolia), 5 drops Roman Chamomile Essential Oil (Chamaemelum nobile), 2 drops Vetiver Essential Oil (Vetiveria zizanioides), 30ml Jojoba Carrier Oil (Simmondsia chinensis)

Process: In a dark glass bottle, combine Lavender, Roman Chamomile, and Vetiver essential oils. Add Jojoba carrier oil to dilute. Shake gently to blend. Apply to wrists and temples before bedtime.

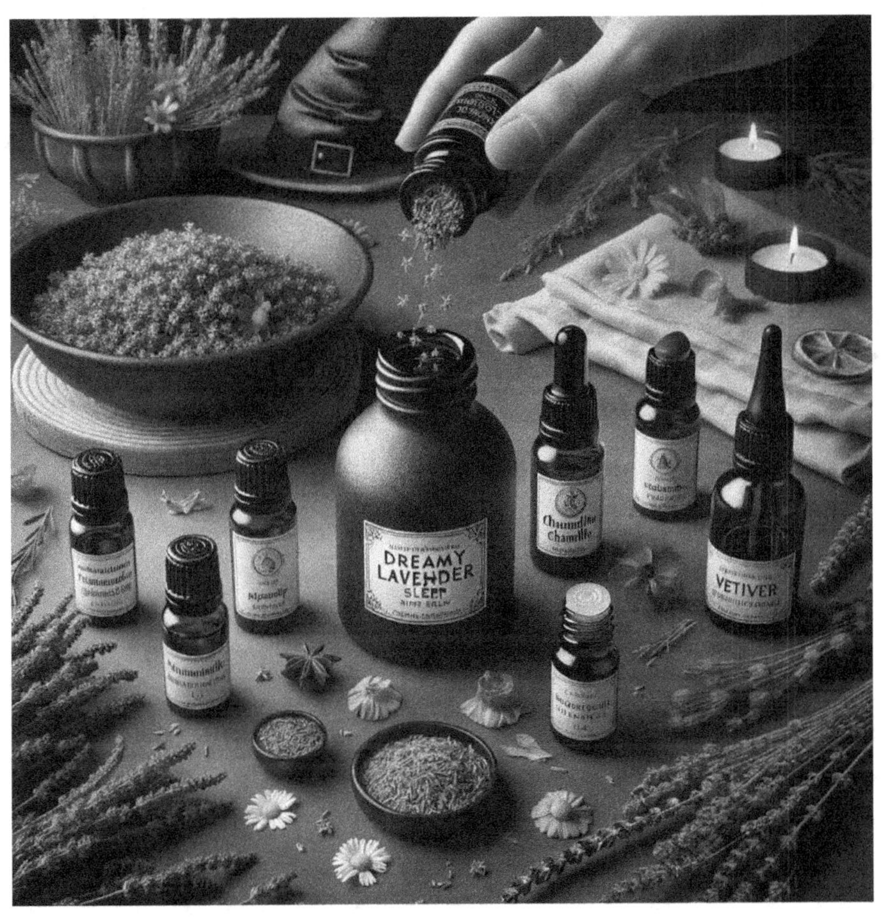

Citrus Focus Enhancer

P.T.: 3 minutes

Ingr.: 7 drops Lemon Essential Oil (Citrus limon), 5 drops Rosemary Essential Oil (Rosmarinus officinalis), 3 drops Peppermint Essential Oil (Mentha piperita), Diffuser

Process: Add Lemon, Rosemary, and Peppermint essential oils to the diffuser with water. Use during work or study sessions to enhance concentration.

Energizing Morning Mist

P.T.: 5 minutes

Ingr.: 8 drops Grapefruit Essential Oil (Citrus paradisi), 4 drops Ginger Essential Oil (Zingiber officinale), 100ml distilled water, Spray bottle

Process: Mix Grapefruit and Ginger essential oils with distilled water in a spray bottle. Shake well. Spritz around your living space in the morning for an energizing atmosphere.

Soothing Sleep Pillow Spray

P.T.: 4 minutes

Ingr.: 6 drops Cedarwood Essential Oil (Cedrus atlantica), 4 drops Bergamot Essential Oil (Citrus bergamia), 100ml distilled water, 1 tsp Witch Hazel (Hamamelis virginiana), Spray bottle

Process: Combine Cedarwood and Bergamot essential oils with witch hazel in a spray bottle. Add distilled water and shake well. Mist over pillows and bed linens before sleep.

Midday Energy Booster Roll-On

P.T.: 5 minutes

Ingr.: 5 drops Eucalyptus Essential Oil (Eucalyptus globulus), 5 drops Sweet Orange Essential Oil (Citrus sinensis), 10ml Fractionated Coconut Oil (Cocos nucifera), Roll-on bottle

Process: In a roll-on bottle, mix Eucalyptus and Sweet Orange essential oils with Fractionated Coconut Oil. Shake well to blend. Apply to pulse points for a quick midday energy boost.

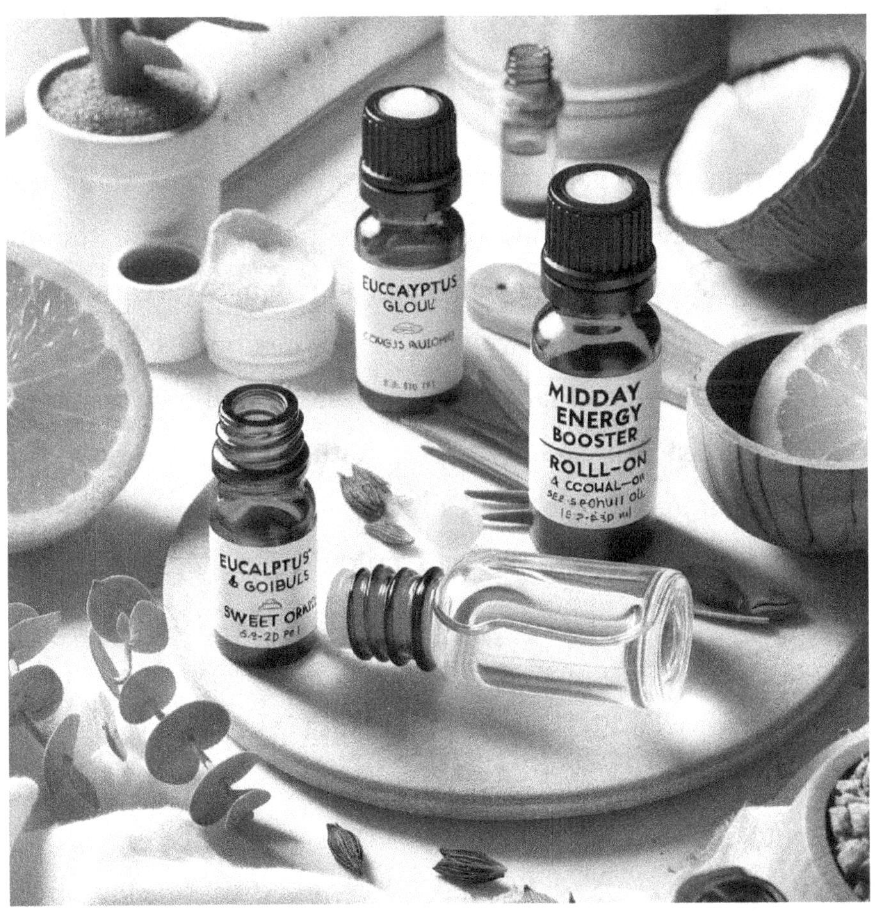

DIY Natural Cleaning Solutions with Essential Oils

In the modern quest for a healthier lifestyle and a greener planet, incorporating essential oils into DIY natural cleaning solutions is a transformative step. This practice not only harnesses the potent antimicrobial properties of essential oils but also infuses daily chores with delightful fragrances, turning routine tasks into sensorial experiences. The art of creating these natural cleaning agents is not just an exercise in sustainability; it is an expression of care for our homes and the environment.

The journey into making your own natural cleaning solutions begins with understanding the natural properties of essential oils. Oils like tea tree, eucalyptus, and lemon are not just celebrated for their invigorating scents; they possess powerful cleansing properties that make them ideal for home cleaning solutions. Tea tree oil, with its natural antibacterial and antifungal qualities, becomes a formidable ingredient in combating household mold and mildew. Eucalyptus, known for its antiseptic properties, is perfect for wiping down surfaces in bathrooms and kitchens. Lemon oil, with its natural acidity and refreshing scent, shines in cutting through grease and grime.

Creating an all-purpose cleaner is a simple yet rewarding endeavor. In a spray bottle, mix distilled water with white vinegar, an age-old cleaning agent. Add a generous helping of lemon oil for its degreasing properties and a touch of lavender for its soothing aroma and antibacterial qualities. This concoction not only cleans effectively but also leaves a fresh, uplifting scent that revitalizes the space.

For a natural glass cleaner, the clarity of the solution is mirrored in its ingredients. Combine distilled water with white vinegar, a staple in natural cleaning for its streak-free shine. Add a few drops of peppermint oil for its crisp, invigorating scent and its ability to dissuade spiders and insects from making homes near windows. The result is a cleaning solution that leaves windows and mirrors sparkling, imbued with a refreshing fragrance.

In the realm of floor cleaning, essential oils offer not just cleanliness but also an aromatic treat. A simple floor cleaner can be crafted by blending hot water with a dash of liquid castile soap, renowned for its gentle yet effective cleansing properties. Adding orange oil can elevate this solution; its citrusy aroma energizes the space while its cleaning properties leave floors spotless and inviting.

Transforming the laundry routine is another area where essential oils shine. Adding a few drops of eucalyptus or lavender oil to unscented laundry detergent can impart a subtle, pleasant aroma to clothes while offering their antimicrobial benefits. For a natural fabric softener, white vinegar can be used in place of commercial products, with a few drops of your favorite essential oil to infuse clothes with a gentle, natural fragrance.

In crafting these DIY solutions, the choice of essential oils can be tailored to personal preferences and specific cleaning needs. It's an opportunity to experiment with different scents and properties, discovering combinations that resonate both with the task at hand and the desired ambiance.

Embracing DIY natural cleaning solutions with essential oils is more than a choice for eco-friendly living; it is a celebration of nature's gifts and a commitment to a healthier lifestyle. These homemade concoctions are a testament to the power of nature's simplicity, effectiveness, and beauty. They transform the mundane into the delightful, infusing everyday cleaning routines with joy and satisfaction, all while ensuring the well-being of our homes and our planet.

Book 2: Aromatic Remedies: Therapeutic Applications of Essential Oils

CHAPTER 1: Holistic Healing with Essential Oils

Venturing into the world of holistic healing with essential oils opens a gateway to discovering the profound effects these natural elixirs have on our well-being. We navigate the diverse landscape of aromatherapy, where each drop of essential oil is a key to enhanced health and wellness. From easing stress and pain to bolstering the immune system, essential oils reveal their versatility and potency as allies in health. They bridge traditional healing practices with contemporary wellness, highlighting nature's capacity to nurture and heal. Delving into the therapeutic benefits of essential oils, we learn to integrate their natural power into our daily lives, fostering a balanced and healthy existence.

Aromatherapy for Stress Relief and Relaxation

In the bustling rhythm of modern life, the quest for stress relief and relaxation has become paramount. Aromatherapy, a centuries-old practice, emerges as a beacon of solace, offering natural, holistic ways to alleviate stress and foster relaxation. This ancient art, harnessing the essence of plants through their essential oils, interacts with our bodies in a way that transcends the mere sense of smell, touching the very core of our well-being.

At the heart of aromatherapy's power for stress relief is its ability to interact with the limbic system, the brain's emotional center. When we inhale the aroma of essential oils, molecules enter the nostrils and drift up to the olfactory receptors. This olfactory input then triggers the limbic system, influencing emotions, mood, and memory. Essential oils like lavender, renowned for their calming properties, can reduce cortisol levels, the body's stress hormone, ushering in a sense of peace and calm.

The process of using essential oils for stress relief is both an art and a science. Lavender, with its sweet, floral aroma, is a cornerstone in stress-relief aromatherapy. Studies have shown that lavender oil can significantly decrease anxiety and improve mood. It can be used in various ways: diffused in the air during a stressful workday, added to a warm bath in the evening, or applied topically, diluted in a carrier oil, for a calming massage.

Another essential oil, Bergamot, with its citrusy yet slightly floral fragrance, is a mood enhancer and stress reliever. Unlike other citrus oils that energize, Bergamot is known for its unique ability to uplift yet relax, making it ideal for balancing mood swings associated with stress.

Ylang Ylang, a tropical flower's oil, is celebrated for its rich, sweet aroma and is often used in reducing stress and promoting relaxation. Its efficacy lies in its ability to decrease heart rate and soothe the nervous system, creating a tranquil environment for the mind and body.

Roman Chamomile, with its light, apple-like scent, is a gentle yet potent relaxant, often used in aromatherapy to ease irritability and nervous tension. When inhaled or applied topically, it can help soothe the mind and relax the muscles, promoting a sense of serenity.

The practice of blending these oils can enhance their stress-relieving properties. For instance, combining Lavender and Bergamot creates a synergy that is both calming and uplifting, ideal for times when stress is high, but energy must be maintained.

The method of application also plays a significant role in how these oils impart their benefits. Diffusion is a popular method, dispersing the oil's molecules into the air for inhalation. This method can create an ambient atmosphere of calm throughout a space. For a more direct approach, topical application of diluted essential oils in massages can work wonders in alleviating stress-related muscle tension.

In addition to these methods, creating a personal aromatherapy inhaler with a blend of stress-relieving oils can provide on-the-go relief. This portable solution allows for immediate response to stressful situations, providing a quick and discreet way to achieve relaxation.

Aromatherapy for stress relief and relaxation is not just about combating existing stress; it's about creating a proactive routine that incorporates these natural essences into daily life. This practice encourages a holistic approach to managing stress, combining the healing power of nature with mindful self-care, leading to a more balanced, relaxed state of being. In embracing aromatherapy, we open ourselves to a world where relaxation is a natural, integral part of life, and stress, while inevitable, is manageable and transient.

Pain Management and Relief with Essential Oils

In the realm of holistic healing, essential oils emerge as powerful allies in the journey towards managing and alleviating pain. These natural treasures, distilled from plants, embody a synergy of therapeutic properties that offer a multi-dimensional approach to pain relief. They work not only at the physical level, addressing various pain types, but also cater to the emotional components often associated with discomfort.

Among the diverse array of essential oils, ginger oil (Zingiber officinale) is renowned for its efficacy in soothing muscular and arthritic pain. Its key compound, gingerol, has been researched for its anti-inflammatory and pain-relieving qualities. The warming sensation it provides upon topical application can be deeply comforting for sore muscles and inflamed joints.

Peppermint oil (Mentha piperita), with its high menthol content, offers a cooling and numbing effect, making it particularly effective for tension headaches and migraines. The uplifting aroma of peppermint also plays a role in mood enhancement, a vital aspect when dealing with chronic pain conditions.

Lavender oil (Lavandula angustifolia) is a versatile player in pain relief, especially beneficial for nerve-related discomfort. Its calming properties not only reduce inflammation but also help in tempering pain signals, offering relief in conditions like sciatica or neuropathy.

Eucalyptus oil (Eucalyptus globulus) is another essential oil that stands out for its pain-relieving properties, particularly in joint-related discomforts. The presence of eucalyptol in eucalyptus contributes to its effectiveness in reducing inflammation and pain, providing a refreshing relief for those suffering from rheumatoid arthritis and similar ailments.

Topical application is a key method in employing essential oils for pain relief. Diluting oils like Roman chamomile (Chamaemelum nobile) and marjoram (Origanum majorana) with a carrier oil for massage can offer localized relief in sore areas, effectively soothing muscle and joint pain.

Creating blends of essential oils can enhance the overall effectiveness in pain management. For instance, a combination of rosemary (Rosmarinus officinalis) and clary sage (Salvia sclarea) can be particularly effective for menstrual cramps, providing both analgesic and anti-spasmodic relief when massaged into the lower abdomen.

Incorporating essential oils into a warm bath can also offer a holistic pain relief experience. A bath infused with a blend of lavender and eucalyptus oils not only soothes the body but also provides a serene escape, aiding in overall relaxation and pain relief.

While essential oils offer a natural and effective approach to pain management, it's imperative to view them as complementary to medical treatments, not replacements. They are most beneficial when used in conjunction with conventional pain management therapies, providing a natural support system to enhance healing and comfort.

Embracing essential oils in pain management is to embrace nature's wisdom in healing. This natural path not only targets the physical dimensions of pain but also nurtures emotional well-being, offering a comprehensive approach to recovery and comfort. As we explore the potential of these aromatic remedies, we open ourselves to a world of healing where pain relief is intertwined with enhancing the quality of life.

Boosting Immunity with Aromatic Compounds

In the intricate dance of health and wellness, the immune system plays a leading role, guarding our bodies against illnesses and infections. Essential oils, nature's aromatic compounds, emerge as supportive actors in this dance, enhancing the body's natural defense mechanisms through their unique properties. The integration of essential oils into daily routines can provide a significant boost to the immune system, fortifying our health holistically.

At the forefront of immune-boosting essential oils is eucalyptus (Eucalyptus globulus), a potent ally with its strong antiviral and antibacterial properties. The compound 1,8-cineole, prevalent in eucalyptus, is known for its ability to support respiratory health, a vital aspect of immune function. Inhaling eucalyptus oil can help clear nasal passages, protect against respiratory infections, and enhance overall breathing quality.

Tea tree oil (Melaleuca alternifolia) stands out for its remarkable antiseptic qualities. Its broad-spectrum antimicrobial activity makes it a valuable tool in warding off pathogens and supporting the body's immune response. Employing tea tree oil in diffusers or in household cleaning solutions can help purify the environment, reducing the risk of pathogen transmission.

Lemon oil (Citrus limon), with its high vitamin C content, is more than just a refreshing scent. Its antiviral and antibacterial properties make it a natural immune booster.

Lemon oil can stimulate white blood cell production, fortifying the body's defense against infections. Additionally, its uplifting aroma can invigorate the spirit and contribute to overall well-being, an essential component of a strong immune system.

Frankincense oil (Boswellia carterii), often revered as the 'king of oils', has a history of promoting health and longevity. It is known for its anti-inflammatory properties and its ability to support and enhance the immune system. Frankincense oil can be particularly beneficial in reducing the risk of inflammation-related illnesses, a common challenge for the immune system.

The art of blending these oils can create synergistic effects, enhancing their immune-boosting properties. A blend of lavender (Lavandula angustifolia), known for its calming properties, with lemon and tea tree oil can provide a balanced approach to strengthening immunity. This combination not only fortifies the body against pathogens but also supports stress reduction, a crucial factor in maintaining a healthy immune response.

The method of application is key in optimizing the benefits of these oils. Diffusing is a popular and effective way to disperse these immune-boosting aromas into the air, creating an environment conducive to health. Topical application, particularly with carrier oils, can also be effective, especially when massaging areas like the feet or the back of the neck, which are key points in the body's immune system.

Incorporating these essential oils into daily routines, such as adding lemon oil to a morning tea or using eucalyptus oil in a shower steam, can make immune support a natural and enjoyable part of life. This proactive approach to wellness allows essential oils to work in harmony with the body, enhancing its natural defenses.

In adopting essential oils for immune support, it's essential to recognize them as part of a broader health strategy. While they offer significant benefits, they are most effective when combined with a healthy lifestyle, including adequate sleep, nutrition, and exercise.

Embracing essential oils for immune boosting is to embrace a holistic approach to health. It's an acknowledgment of the power of natural remedies and their role in supporting the body's innate healing abilities. As we integrate these aromatic compounds into our lives, we open ourselves to a world of natural wellness, where the body's defenses are not just protected but also nurtured and strengthened.

CHAPTER 2: Mind and Mood Enhancements

In the realm of essential oils, there exists a profound ability to influence and enhance our mental and emotional states.

Essential Oils for Anxiety and Depression

Serenity Now Inhaler Blend

P.T.: 3 minutes

Ingr.: 5 drops Lavender Oil (Lavandula angustifolia), 3 drops Clary Sage Oil (Salvia sclarea), 2 drops Ylang Ylang Oil (Cananga odorata), Aromatherapy inhaler

Process: Add Lavender, Clary Sage, and Ylang Ylang oils to the cotton wick of the inhaler. Assemble the inhaler and use for instant relief during anxious moments.

Calm Mind Diffuser Blend

P.T.: 2 minutes

Ingr.: 4 drops Bergamot Oil (Citrus bergamia), 3 drops Frankincense Oil (Boswellia carterii), 3 drops Sandalwood Oil (Santalum album), Diffuser

Process: Combine Bergamot, Frankincense, and Sandalwood oils in a diffuser with water. Use in living spaces to create a calm, soothing environment.

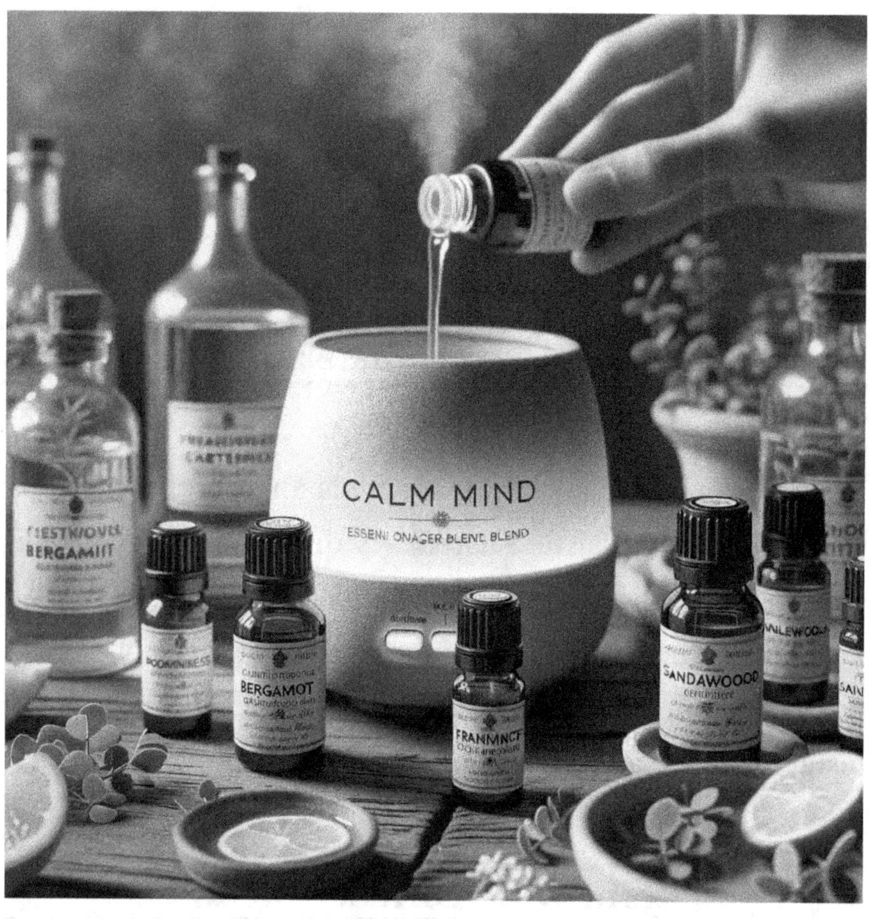

Soothing Bath Elixir

P.T.: 5 minutes

Ingr.: 6 drops Roman Chamomile Oil (Chamaemelum nobile), 4 drops Geranium Oil (Pelargonium graveolens), 100ml Epsom Salts, 30ml Jojoba Carrier Oil

Process: Mix Roman Chamomile and Geranium oils with Jojoba Carrier Oil and Epsom Salts. Add to a warm bath for a relaxing and mood-lifting soak.

Peaceful Slumber Roll-On

P.T.: 4 minutes

Ingr.: 5 drops Sweet Marjoram Oil (Origanum majorana), 5 drops Cedarwood Oil (Cedrus atlantica), 10ml Fractionated Coconut Oil, Roll-on bottle

Process: Blend Sweet Marjoram and Cedarwood oils with Fractionated Coconut Oil in a roll-on bottle. Apply to temples and wrists before bed to ease into a peaceful sleep.

Uplifting Aromatic Spray

P.T.: 5 minutes

Ingr.: 7 drops Sweet Orange Oil (Citrus sinensis), 3 drops Patchouli Oil (Pogostemon cablin), 100ml distilled water, 1 tsp Witch Hazel, Spray bottle

Process: Combine Sweet Orange and Patchouli oils with witch hazel in a spray bottle. Add distilled water and shake well. Use as a room spray to uplift mood and alleviate feelings of depression.

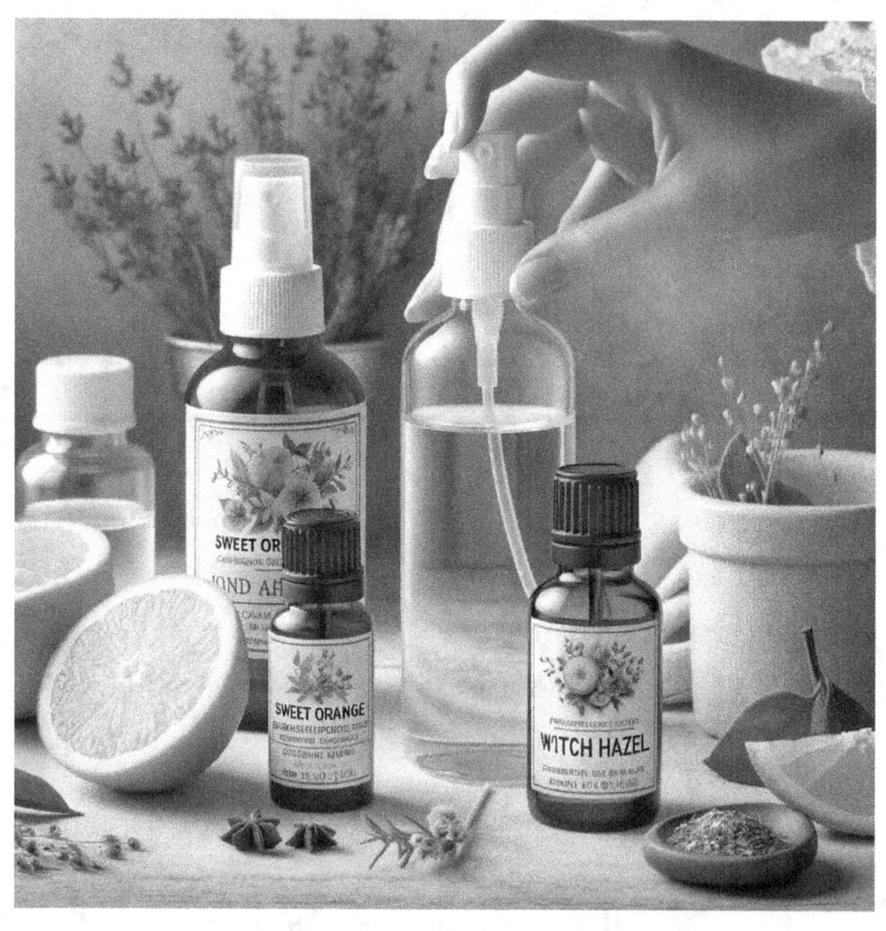

Uplifting Scents: Citrus and Floral Oils

Morning Sunshine Diffuser Blend

P.T.: 2 minutes

Ingr.: 4 drops Grapefruit Oil (Citrus paradisi), 3 drops Jasmine Absolute (Jasminum officinale), 2 drops Lemon Oil (Citrus limon), Diffuser

Process: Add Grapefruit, Jasmine, and Lemon oils to a diffuser filled with water. Use in the morning to invigorate and uplift the mood for a positive start to the day.

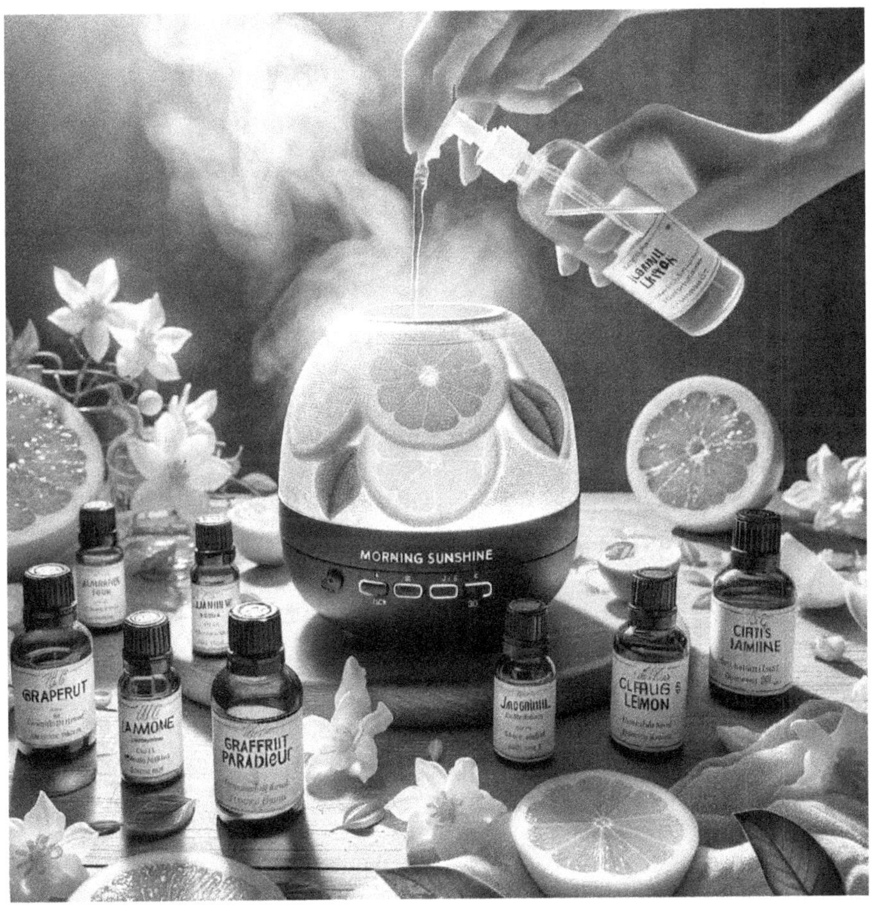

Floral Bliss Room Spray

P.T.: 5 minutes

Ingr.: 6 drops Neroli Oil (Citrus aurantium), 4 drops Rose Oil (Rosa damascena), 100ml distilled water, 1 tsp Ethanol, Spray bottle

Process: Combine Neroli and Rose oils with ethanol in a spray bottle. Add distilled water and shake well. Use as a room spray for an instant mood-lifting and refreshing atmosphere.

Citrus Garden Bath Salts

P.T.: 7 minutes

Ingr.: 5 drops Bergamot Oil (Citrus bergamia), 3 drops Geranium Oil (Pelargonium graveolens), 200g Epsom Salts, 50ml Fractionated Coconut Oil

Process: Mix Bergamot and Geranium oils with Fractionated Coconut Oil. Blend with Epsom Salts thoroughly. Add to a warm bath for an uplifting and rejuvenating experience.

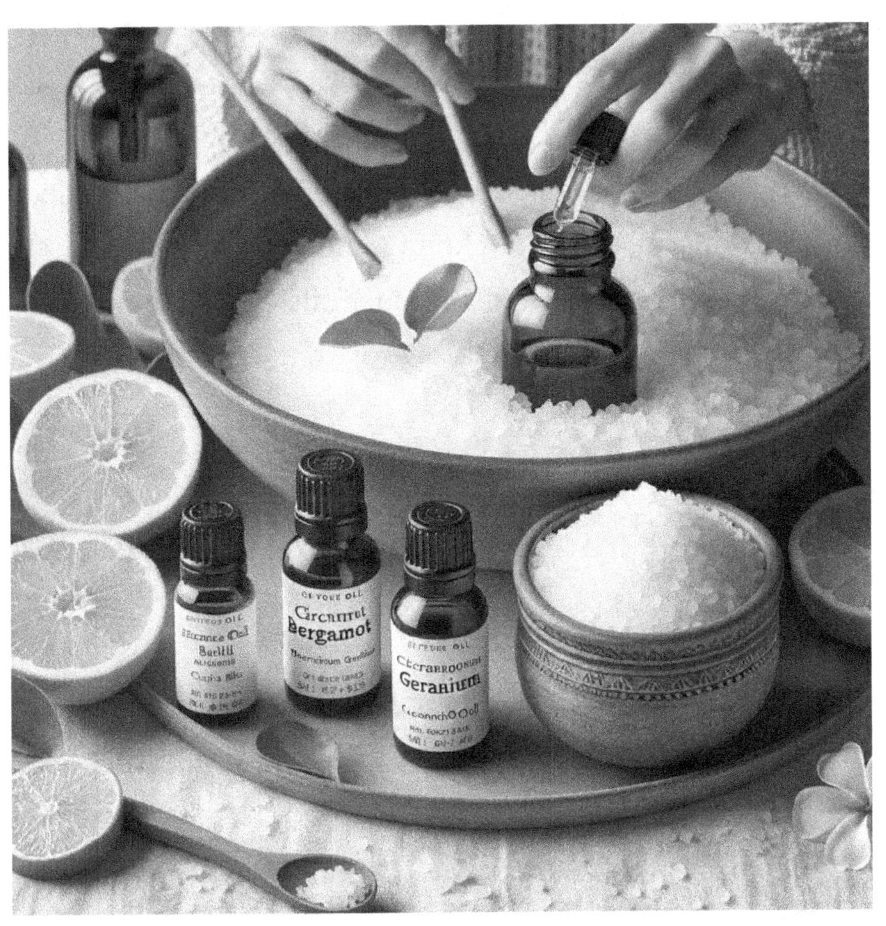

Joyful Pulse Point Roll-On

P.T.: 4 minutes

Ingr.: 4 drops Sweet Orange Oil (Citrus sinensis), 4 drops Ylang Ylang Oil (Cananga odorata), 10ml Jojoba Oil, Roll-on bottle

Process: Blend Sweet Orange and Ylang Ylang oils with Jojoba Oil in a roll-on bottle. Apply to pulse points such as wrists and neck whenever in need of an emotional lift.

Energizing Massage Oil

P.T.: 6 minutes

Ingr.: 6 drops Lime Oil (Citrus aurantifolia), 4 drops Lavender Oil (Lavandula angustifolia), 30ml Almond Oil

Process: Combine Lime and Lavender oils with Almond Oil in a small container. Use as a massage oil to invigorate the senses and boost energy levels.

Grounding and Calming: Woods and Resins

Forest Embrace Diffuser Blend

P.T.: 2 minutes

Ingr.: 5 drops Cedarwood Oil (Cedrus atlantica), 4 drops Sandalwood Oil (Santalum album), 3 drops Frankincense Oil (Boswellia carterii), Diffuser

Process: Add Cedarwood, Sandalwood, and Frankincense oils to a diffuser filled with water. Use to create a grounding and calming atmosphere, reminiscent of a walk through a serene forest.

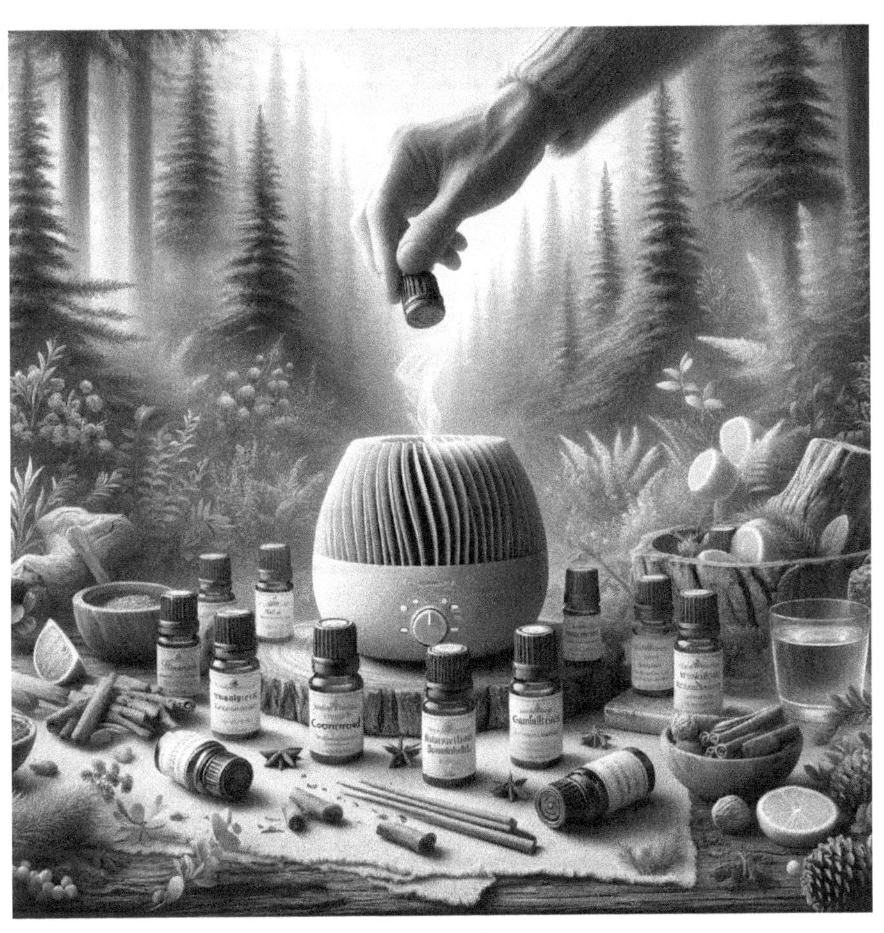

Earthy Tranquility Roller

P.T.: 3 minutes

Ingr.: 6 drops Vetiver Oil (Vetiveria zizanioides), 4 drops Patchouli Oil (Pogostemon cablin), 10ml Grapeseed Oil, Roll-on bottle

Process: Combine Vetiver and Patchouli oils with Grapeseed Oil in a roll-on bottle. Apply to the wrists and temples for grounding and tranquility during stressful moments.

Resin Relaxation Bath Oil

P.T.: 5 minutes

Ingr.: 5 drops Myrrh Oil (Commiphora myrrha), 5 drops Pine Oil (Pinus sylvestris), 30ml Sweet Almond Oil, 1 tbsp Milk

Process: Mix Myrrh and Pine oils with Sweet Almond Oil and milk. Add to a warm bath for a deeply calming and grounding experience.

Soothing Sleep Pillow Mist

P.T.: 4 minutes

Ingr.: 7 drops Balsam Fir Oil (Abies balsamea), 3 drops Copaiba Balsam Oil (Copaifera officinalis), 100ml distilled water, 1 tsp Witch Hazel, Spray bottle

Process: Blend Balsam Fir and Copaiba Balsam oils with witch hazel in a spray bottle. Add distilled water and shake well. Mist over pillows and bed linens for a restful and grounding night's sleep.

Meditation Anointing Oil

P.T.: 5 minutes

Ingr.: 4 drops Palo Santo Oil (Bursera graveolens), 4 drops Frankincense Oil (Boswellia carterii), 20ml Jojoba Oil, Small vial or container

Process: Mix Palo Santo and Frankincense oils with Jojoba Oil in a small container. Use to anoint the forehead and wrists before meditation for enhanced grounding and spiritual connection.

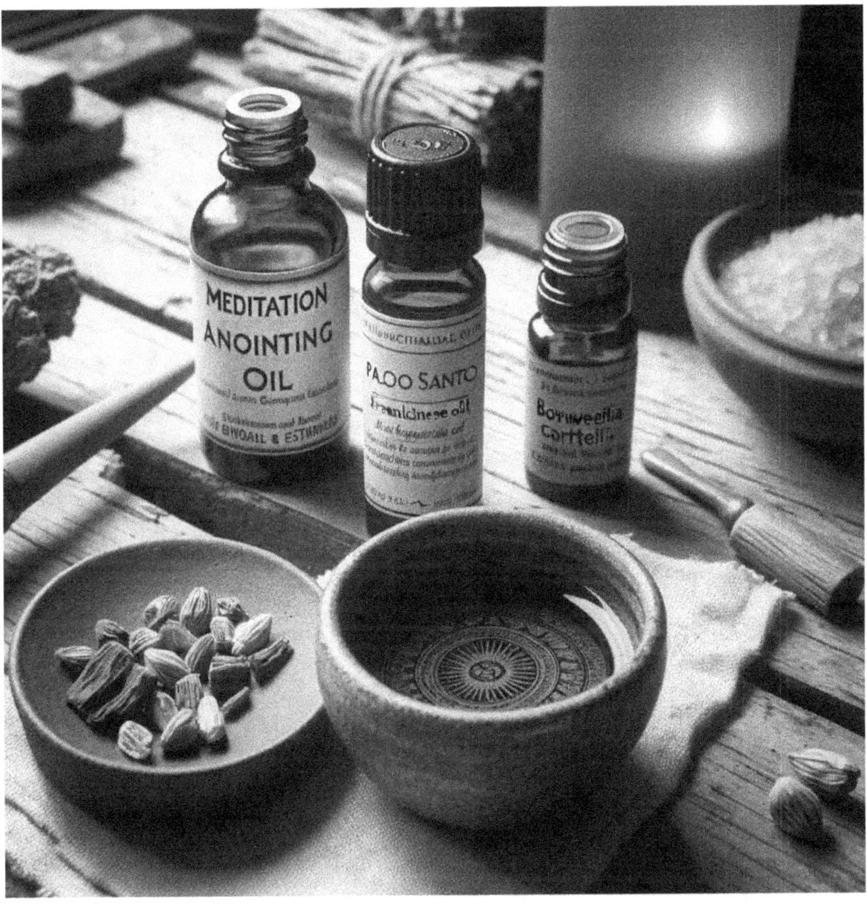

As we conclude our exploration of mind and mood enhancements through essential oils, we gain an enriched understanding of their capacity to harmonize and elevate our emotional states. From soothing the complexities of anxiety and depression to invigorating the soul with uplifting scents, the journey has been illuminating. We've also embraced the stabilizing influence of woody and resinous oils, grounding ourselves amidst life's fluctuations. This exploration highlights the inherent power of nature's essences in positively influencing our emotional well-being. Integrating these natural wonders into our daily practices allows us to embrace a holistic approach to emotional health, tapping into the nurturing power of aromatherapy to care for our minds and hearts.

CHAPTER 3: Physical Wellness and Aromatherapy

Embarking on a journey through the world of physical wellness and aromatherapy, we explore the remarkable abilities of essential oils to nurture the body's health.

Essential Oils in Digestive Health

The journey of maintaining and enhancing digestive health finds a natural and efficacious ally in the world of aromatherapy. Essential oils, with their potent and diverse therapeutic properties, offer a unique approach to supporting digestive wellness. This exploration delves into how these aromatic extracts can be integrated into practices for promoting a healthy and balanced digestive system.

At the forefront of digestive health in aromatherapy are essential oils known for their carminative and antispasmodic properties. Peppermint oil (Mentha piperita) is a prime example, revered for its ability to ease digestive discomforts like bloating and gas. The key component, menthol, aids in relaxing the smooth muscles of the gastrointestinal tract, thereby alleviating cramps and spasms. A simple inhalation of peppermint oil or a gentle abdominal massage using a blend of peppermint oil and a carrier can provide quick relief.

Ginger oil (Zingiber officinale), extracted from the root of the ginger plant, is another powerhouse for digestive health. Known for its warming and anti-inflammatory properties, ginger oil can be beneficial in soothing digestive upset, particularly nausea. Its efficacy in reducing symptoms of motion sickness and morning sickness has been well documented. A warm compress using diluted ginger oil or inhaling its strong, spicy aroma can help in settling digestive turmoil.

Fennel oil (Foeniculum vulgare), with its sweet, licorice-like aroma, is traditionally used for its supportive role in digestion. It's particularly effective in combating flatulence and encouraging healthy digestion. Fennel oil's gentle yet potent nature makes it suitable for soothing minor digestive ailments. Blending fennel oil with a carrier oil for abdominal massages can stimulate the digestive system and ease discomfort.

Lemon oil (Citrus limon) is celebrated not only for its refreshing scent but also for its ability to detoxify and cleanse. Its natural antioxidant and anti-inflammatory properties make it an excellent choice for supporting liver health and aiding digestion. Adding a drop of lemon oil to a glass of water in the morning can stimulate the digestive system and kick-start metabolism, offering a refreshing and healthful start to the day.

An often overlooked aspect of digestive health is the emotional connection to our gastrointestinal system. Stress and anxiety can significantly impact digestion, leading to issues like irritable bowel syndrome (IBS). Lavender oil (Lavandula angustifolia), known for its calming effects, can be a valuable tool in managing stress-related digestive problems. Using lavender oil in a diffuser or as part of a relaxing evening routine can help reduce stress, thus positively impacting digestive health.

Incorporating these essential oils into daily routines requires a balanced and informed approach. While essential oils offer considerable benefits for digestive health, they are not a substitute for medical advice or treatment. They work best as a complementary approach, offering natural support alongside other health practices.

In embracing essential oils for digestive health, we open ourselves to a holistic approach to wellness. This natural path not only targets specific digestive issues but also considers the intricate connection between our gut, mind, and overall health. As we integrate these aromatic treasures into our wellness journey, we embrace the harmonious balance they bring to our digestive health, enhancing our overall quality of life through nature's own healing essence.

Respiratory Support and Essential Oils

In the pursuit of physical wellness, maintaining a healthy respiratory system is paramount. The lungs, our vital organs of breath, are not only essential for life but also a reflection of our overall health. In this context, essential oils, with their diverse and potent therapeutic properties, emerge as valuable allies for respiratory support. These natural essences, extracted from plants, offer a holistic approach to nurturing and maintaining respiratory health.

The efficacy of essential oils in respiratory care lies in their ability to provide relief, clear airways, and support the body's natural healing processes. Eucalyptus oil (Eucalyptus globulus), with its high concentration of 1,8-cineole, is renowned for its decongestant properties. This powerful compound helps to break up mucus and clear congestion, making eucalyptus oil a go-to remedy for conditions like colds, coughs, and sinusitis. Inhaling eucalyptus oil, either through a diffuser or by adding a few drops to a steamy shower, can provide immediate relief by opening up the nasal passages and bronchial tubes.

Peppermint oil (Mentha piperita) is another potent respiratory aid. Its main component, menthol, is effective in soothing sore throats and easing breathing difficulties. The cooling sensation it provides can be particularly soothing during episodes of cough or throat irritation. A simple inhalation of peppermint oil or using it in a throat gargle can offer quick relief.

Another essential oil that plays a significant role in respiratory health is tea tree oil (Melaleuca alternifolia). Known for its antimicrobial properties, tea tree oil can help fight infections that affect the respiratory system. Its ability to support the immune system makes it an excellent choice for preventive care. Using tea tree oil in a diffuser or as part of a chest rub (diluted with a carrier oil) can help in keeping the respiratory system healthy.

Thyme oil (Thymus vulgaris) is a lesser-known yet powerful oil for respiratory support. Rich in thymol, it has strong antibacterial and antiviral properties, making it effective in treating respiratory infections. Thyme oil can be particularly beneficial for bronchitis and other lower respiratory tract infections. Inhalation or topical application (when diluted) of thyme oil can help in alleviating symptoms and speeding up recovery.

Lavender oil (Lavandula angustifolia), widely known for its calming properties, also plays a role in respiratory health. Its anti-inflammatory properties can help reduce swelling in the respiratory tract, making breathing easier. Additionally, its soothing effect can help reduce anxiety and stress, which are often exacerbated during respiratory distress.

Incorporating these essential oils into daily routines for respiratory support can involve various methods. Diffusing oils throughout the home, especially during the cold and flu season, can help purify the air and prevent the spread of airborne pathogens. Creating a chest rub using a blend of eucalyptus, peppermint, and lavender oils diluted in a carrier oil like coconut oil can provide soothing relief. For those who prefer a more direct method, steam inhalation with a few drops of eucalyptus or peppermint oil can be highly effective.

While essential oils offer significant benefits for respiratory health, it's important to use them responsibly. Individuals with asthma or other respiratory conditions should consult with a healthcare provider before using essential oils, as they can sometimes trigger allergic reactions or interact with medications.

In embracing essential oils for respiratory support, we tap into the ancient wisdom of natural healing, utilizing the power of plants to support our body's vital breath. This holistic approach not only targets the symptoms but also considers the overall health of the respiratory system, offering a path to enhanced wellness and vitality. As we integrate these natural remedies into our lives, we breathe easier, knowing we are nurturing our bodies with the healing essence of nature.

Skin Care: Healing with Essential Oils

In the realm of physical wellness, the health of our skin is not just a matter of beauty, but also a reflection of our overall well-being. Essential oils, with their myriad of therapeutic properties, offer a natural and effective approach to skin care, transcending conventional beauty routines.

Essential oils for skin care are chosen for their specific benefits, such as anti-inflammatory, antibacterial, moisturizing, or regenerative properties. Lavender oil (Lavandula angustifolia) is a quintessential example, renowned for its soothing and healing properties. Ideal for all skin types, it can calm inflammation, speed up wound healing, and even provide relief from skin conditions like eczema and psoriasis. A few drops of lavender oil added to a carrier oil or lotion can create a simple yet effective remedy for irritated or sensitive skin.

Tea tree oil (Melaleuca alternifolia) is a powerhouse for acne-prone skin, thanks to its antibacterial and antiseptic properties. It can combat acne-causing bacteria, reduce inflammation, and help prevent future breakouts. When diluted properly, tea tree oil can be applied directly to blemishes or mixed into cleansers and toners for a more comprehensive acne-fighting regimen.

For aging skin, frankincense oil (Boswellia carterii) is a valuable ally. Its ability to promote cell regeneration and protect existing cells makes it an excellent choice for reducing the appearance of wrinkles and fine lines. Frankincense oil, blended with a nourishing carrier oil like jojoba or rosehip, can be a luxurious, anti-aging facial serum.

Rose oil (Rosa damascena), with its exquisite fragrance and potent skin-enhancing properties, is a treasure in skin care. Known for its hydrating and toning effects, rose oil can help improve skin texture, add radiance, and maintain the skin's pH balance. Its anti-inflammatory qualities also make it suitable for calming redness and irritation.

For those with oily or combination skin, geranium oil (Pelargonium graveolens) can be particularly beneficial. Its astringent properties help tighten and tone the skin, reducing excess oiliness, while its balancing effect can help regulate the skin's natural oil production. A facial mist or toner incorporating geranium oil can be a refreshing addition to the skin care routine.

Incorporating these essential oils into skin care requires a thoughtful and tailored approach. Essential oils should always be diluted with a suitable carrier oil or skin care product to avoid irritation. Patch tests are recommended to ensure skin compatibility. Furthermore, understanding one's skin type and concerns is crucial in selecting the right essential oils and formulations.

Beyond individual oil applications, the art of blending essential oils for skin care allows for the creation of custom solutions targeting specific skin concerns. A blend of chamomile (Matricaria chamomilla) and calendula (Calendula officinalis) oils, for instance, can be wonderfully soothing for sensitive skin. Such blends, when incorporated into daily skin care routines, can lead to significant improvements in skin health and appearance.

Essential oils in skin care are not just about addressing skin issues; they offer an experience that nurtures the skin and senses. They connect us to the rhythms of nature, reminding us that beauty and health are inherently linked. As we embrace these natural essences for our skin, we step into a world where wellness is holistic, where skin care is as much about nourishing the soul as it is about enhancing the skin. This approach to skin care, rooted in the healing power of nature, not only beautifies the skin but also harmonizes our connection with the natural world.

The incorporation of these natural remedies into our wellness practices signifies a commitment to nurturing our bodies with the purity and efficacy of nature. Moving forward, these aromatic treasures stand as allies in our ongoing pursuit of physical health, reminding us of the gentle yet powerful connection we share with the natural world.

CHAPTER 4: Women's Health and Essential Oils

Venturing into the realm of women's health, this chapter unfolds the harmonious relationship between essential oils and the unique aspects of feminine well-being. We explore the nurturing role these natural essences play in balancing hormones, providing comfort during menstrual cycles, and supporting women through the transformative stages of pregnancy and postpartum. Essential oils, with their profound therapeutic properties, emerge as gentle yet powerful aids in addressing the specific health needs of women. They offer a holistic approach, blending the ancient wisdom of plant-based healing with modern understanding of women's health. The journey through these pages is an invitation to embrace the natural support of essential oils, enhancing wellness and harmony at every stage of a woman's life.

Hormonal Balance and Essential Oils

In the intricate tapestry of women's health, hormonal balance plays a pivotal role, influencing everything from mood to physical well-being. Essential oils, with their unique molecular structures and potent biological activities, offer a gentle yet effective approach to nurturing hormonal balance.

The harmonizing power of essential oils in regulating hormones lies in their ability to mimic or influence hormonal activity in the body. Clary sage oil (Salvia sclarea), for instance, is renowned for its ability to help balance estrogen levels. Its phytoestrogen components can be particularly beneficial during menopause, easing symptoms like hot flashes and mood swings. Inhaling clary sage oil or applying it topically (when diluted with a carrier oil) to pulse points can be a soothing ritual for women experiencing hormonal fluctuations.

Geranium oil (Pelargonium graveolens), with its floral and sweet aroma, is another ally in hormonal balance. Known for its ability to regulate adrenal cortex activity, geranium oil can help stabilize hormonal levels. Its mood-enhancing properties also make it a valuable oil for combating premenstrual syndrome (PMS) and menopausal anxiety. Blending geranium oil with lavender oil in a diffuser can create a calming and balancing atmosphere, helping to soothe emotional swings associated with hormonal changes.

Fennel oil (Foeniculum vulgare), often used for its digestive benefits, has a hidden talent in supporting hormonal balance. Fennel's natural compounds mimic the estrogen hormone, making it helpful in regulating menstrual cycles and easing menopausal symptoms. A gentle abdominal massage with diluted fennel oil can provide relief from menstrual cramps and help regulate menstrual cycles.

Rose oil (Rosa damascena), the queen of oils, is not just celebrated for its exquisite scent but also for its profound impact on hormonal health. It's known to stimulate the production of hormones like estrogen, which can be beneficial for those with low estrogen levels. Its uplifting and heart-opening qualities also make it a great emotional support during times of hormonal upheaval.

Ylang Ylang oil (Cananga odorata), with its sweet, heady aroma, is a mood stabilizer and an enhancer of sexual well-being. It can be particularly helpful in balancing hormones related to libido and stress. Diffusing ylang ylang oil or adding it to bathwater can create a relaxing and aphrodisiac atmosphere, beneficial for both emotional and hormonal health.

Incorporating these oils into daily routines involves more than just random application. It requires a mindful approach, understanding the specific needs of the body at different times. For instance, using clary sage and geranium during the premenstrual period, and switching to rose and fennel during menopause, can provide targeted hormonal support.

While essential oils offer a natural avenue for hormonal balance, it's important to use them with knowledge and caution. Consulting with a healthcare provider, especially in cases of hormonal disorders or when taking hormonal medications, is crucial. Additionally, understanding the quality and purity of the essential oils used is essential for their effectiveness and safety.

In embracing essential oils for hormonal balance, we tap into the ancient wisdom of plant medicine, utilizing nature's remedies to support the complex hormonal systems in women's bodies. This approach not only addresses physical symptoms but also honors the emotional and spiritual aspects of hormonal health, providing a holistic path to well-being and harmony. As we integrate these natural essences into our wellness practices, we celebrate the power of nature in supporting the unique journey of womanhood.

Aromatherapy for Menstrual Discomfort

The menstrual cycle, a natural part of a woman's life, can often bring with it discomfort and pain that can be both physically and emotionally draining. In the quest for relief, essential oils emerge as a gentle yet potent tool, offering a natural alternative or complement to traditional pain relief methods.

Menstrual discomfort, often characterized by cramps, bloating, and mood swings, can significantly impact daily life. Clary sage oil (Salvia sclarea) is highly esteemed for its antispasmodic properties, making it particularly effective in easing menstrual cramps. Its ability to balance hormones also contributes to its effectiveness in reducing PMS symptoms. A warm compress soaked in a mixture of clary sage oil and a carrier oil, when applied to the lower abdomen, can provide significant relief from cramps.

Lavender oil (Lavandula angustifolia), renowned for its calming and anti-inflammatory properties, is another valuable ally during menstruation. It can help soothe both physical pain and emotional stress often associated with menstrual cycles. Using lavender oil in a bath, or as part of a massage oil blend, can promote relaxation and alleviate discomfort.

Geranium oil (Pelargonium graveolens), with its hormone-balancing and analgesic properties, can be beneficial in managing PMS symptoms and menstrual discomfort. Its uplifting aroma can also help counteract mood swings and irritability. Blending geranium with carrier oils for a soothing abdominal massage can help reduce pain and enhance emotional well-being.

Peppermint oil (Mentha piperita), known for its cooling and analgesic effects, can offer relief from headaches and fatigue related to the menstrual cycle. Its refreshing scent can also help in alleviating nausea and fatigue. A diluted peppermint oil applied to the temples or the back of the neck can provide quick relief from menstrual headaches.

Marjoram oil (Origanum majorana), a lesser-known but highly effective oil for menstrual discomfort, has warming and soothing properties. It can help in relaxing muscle spasms and reducing pain. A warm bath enhanced with marjoram oil can be a comforting remedy for menstrual cramps.

Incorporating these essential oils into a holistic menstrual discomfort management plan involves understanding individual responses and preferences. It's important to consider the intensity of symptoms and personal sensitivity to certain scents when choosing the right oils. For instance, while some may find relief with a warm compress of clary sage, others may prefer the soothing aroma of lavender in a diffuser.

While essential oils offer a natural way to manage menstrual discomfort, it's important to approach them with care. Proper dilution is crucial to avoid skin irritation, and a patch test is recommended before topical application. Additionally, women who are pregnant or have certain medical conditions should consult with a healthcare provider before using essential oils.

In embracing aromatherapy for menstrual discomfort, we connect with the ancient practice of using plant essences for healing. This approach not only addresses the physical aspects of menstrual pain but also considers the emotional and mental well-being, offering a holistic path to comfort and relief. As we integrate these natural remedies into our routines, we honor our bodies' rhythms and cycles, nurturing ourselves with the gentle power of nature's gifts.

Essential Oils for Pregnancy and Postpartum Care

Gentle Belly Massage Oil for Pregnancy

P.T.: 5 minutes

Ingr.: 4 drops Lavender Oil (Lavandula angustifolia), 3 drops Mandarin Oil (Citrus reticulata), 30ml Sweet Almond Oil (Prunus amygdalus dulcis)

Process: Blend Lavender and Mandarin oils with Sweet Almond Oil in a small bottle. Gently massage onto the belly to soothe stretching skin and relax.

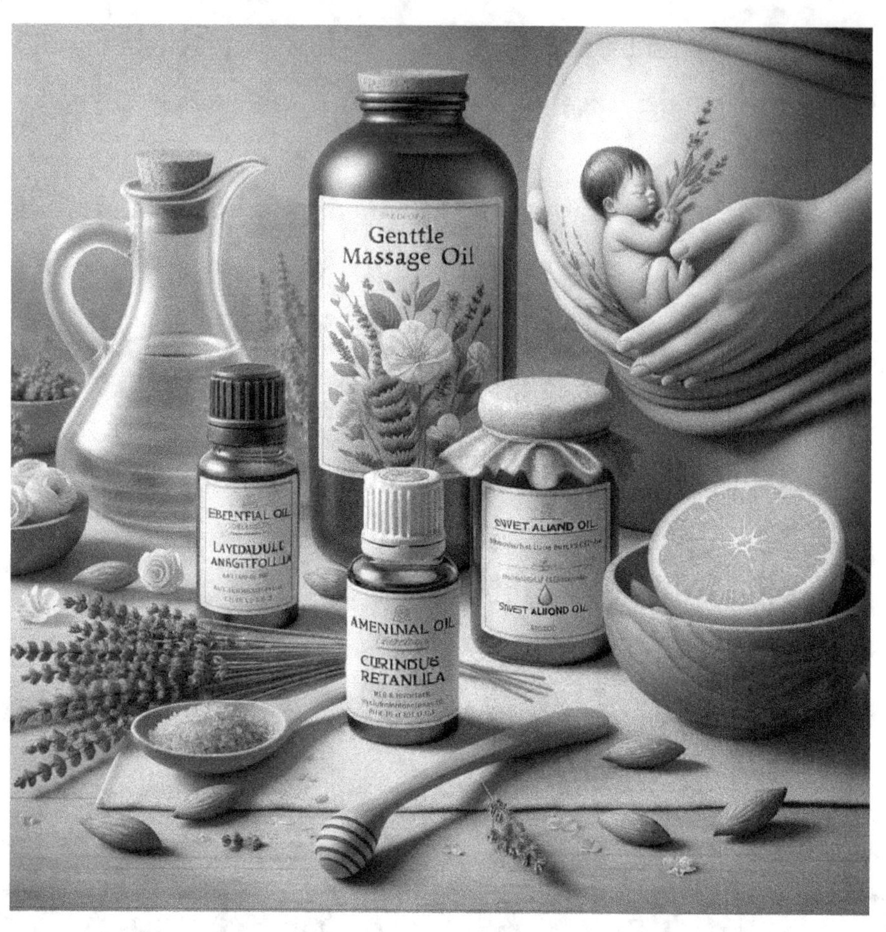

Postpartum Soothing Bath Blend

P.T.: 6 minutes

Ingr.: 5 drops Frankincense Oil (Boswellia carterii), 4 drops Geranium Oil (Pelargonium graveolens), 100ml Epsom Salts, 30ml Fractionated Coconut Oil (Cocos nucifera)

Process: Mix Frankincense and Geranium oils with Fractionated Coconut Oil. Combine with Epsom Salts. Add to a warm bath for postpartum healing and relaxation.

Nurturing Foot Rub for Pregnancy

P.T.: 4 minutes

Ingr.: 5 drops Cypress Oil (Cupressus sempervirens), 4 drops Lemon Oil (Citrus limon), 30ml Grapeseed Oil (Vitis vinifera)

Process: Combine Cypress and Lemon oils with Grapeseed Oil. Use for a gentle foot massage to reduce swelling and discomfort during pregnancy.

Calming Postpartum Diffuser Blend

P.T.: 2 minutes

Ingr.: 3 drops Bergamot Oil (Citrus bergamia), 3 drops Ylang Ylang Oil (Cananga odorata), 2 drops Clary Sage Oil (Salvia sclarea), Diffuser

Process: Add Bergamot, Ylang Ylang, and Clary Sage oils to a diffuser with water. Diffuse in the room for calming postpartum emotions and stress relief.

Stretch Mark Prevention Oil

P.T.: 5 minutes

Ingr.: 4 drops Neroli Oil (Citrus aurantium), 3 drops Rosehip Oil (Rosa canina), 30ml Jojoba Oil (Simmondsia chinensis)

Process: Blend Neroli and Rosehip oils with Jojoba Oil in a bottle. Apply daily to areas prone to stretch marks to nourish and improve skin elasticity during pregnancy.

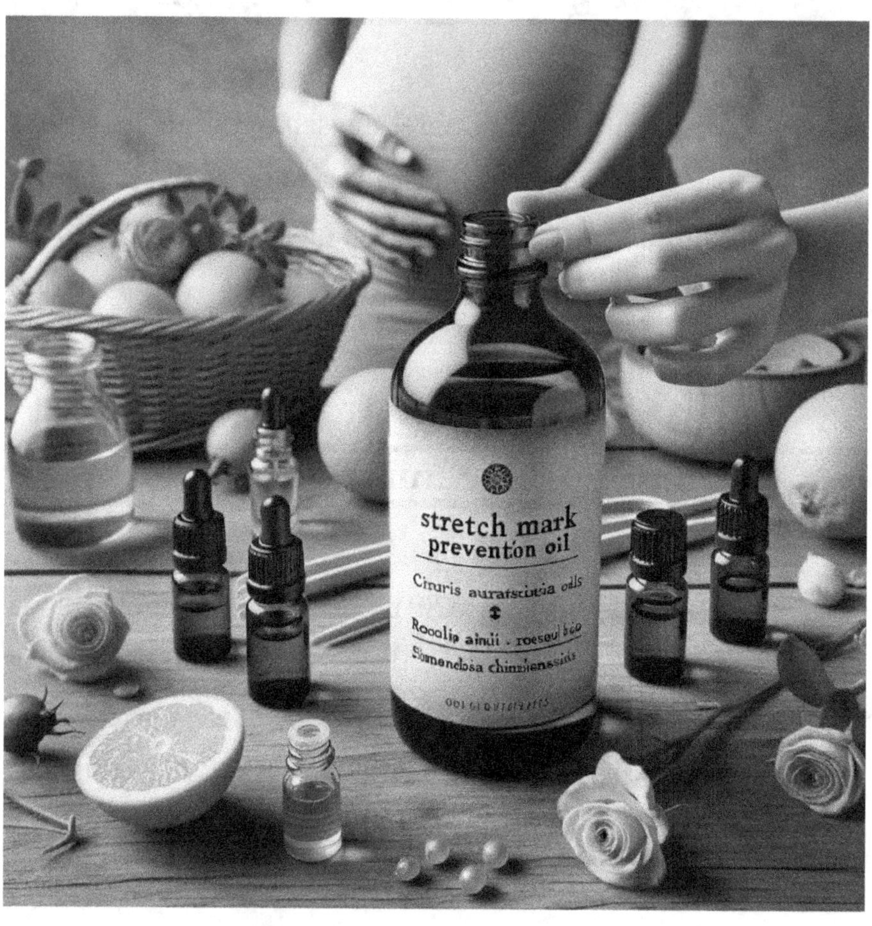

stretch mark
prevention oil

As we conclude our exploration of women's health and essential oils, we carry with us a deeper appreciation of the natural synergy between aromatherapy and the diverse phases of a woman's life. This chapter has illuminated the ways in which essential oils can be integrated into daily routines, offering support and relief from hormonal imbalances, menstrual discomfort, and the challenges of pregnancy and postpartum. We have witnessed the versatility of these aromatic compounds, recognizing their potential not just in physical healing, but also in fostering emotional and mental well-being. Embracing these natural remedies, we acknowledge the power of a holistic approach to health, one that honors the unique needs and experiences of women. As we move forward, these insights guide us to nurture ourselves and others with the gentle, healing touch of nature's essences.

Book 3: Home Apothecary: Essential Oil Recipes for a Natural Lifestyle

CHAPTER 1: Personal Care Potions

Embarking on a journey into the realm of natural self-care, this chapter unveils a treasure trove of essential oil-based recipes for enhancing skin, hair, and oral health. Here, the ancient art of aromatherapy meets modern personal care needs, offering a range of nourishing elixirs, rejuvenating treatments, and purifying blends. Each concoction is a blend of nature's finest, harnessing the therapeutic potency of essential oils and natural ingredients. From revitalizing skin care formulations to hair care treatments that restore luster and strength, and oral care blends for a refreshing clean, these recipes invite you to embrace the elegance and efficacy of nature-driven self-care. This foray into personal care potions is an invitation to nurture the body with nature's purest essences, fostering well-being and natural beauty in harmony with the earth.

Nourishing Skin Care Recipes

Hydrating Rose Facial Serum

P.T.: 10 minutes

Ingr.: 5 drops Rose Oil (Rosa damascena), 4 drops Frankincense Oil (Boswellia carterii), 30ml Argan Oil (Argania spinosa), 10ml Jojoba Oil (Simmondsia chinensis), Glass dropper bottle

Process: In a glass dropper bottle, blend Rose and Frankincense oils with Argan and Jojoba oils. Shake well to combine. Apply a few drops to the face and neck after cleansing for deep hydration.

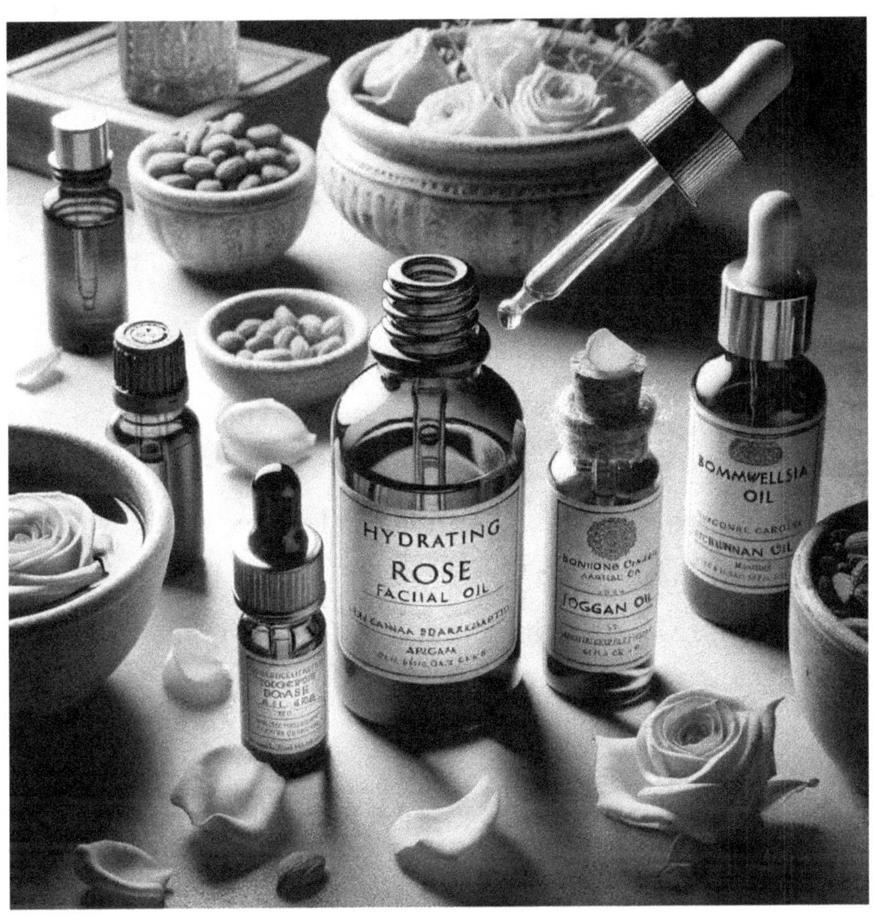

Soothing Chamomile Night Cream

P.T.: 15 minutes

Ingr.: 3 drops Chamomile Oil (Matricaria chamomilla), 2 drops Lavender Oil (Lavandula angustifolia), 30g Shea Butter (Butyrospermum parkii), 20ml Almond Oil (Prunus dulcis), Small jar

Process: Gently melt Shea Butter in a double boiler. Remove from heat and stir in Almond Oil. Once slightly cooled, add

Chamomile and Lavender oils. Transfer to a jar and let it solidify. Use nightly for soothing and nourishing skin.

Antioxidant Green Tea Facial Mist

P.T.: 20 minutes

Ingr.: 4 drops Green Tea Extract, 3 drops Neroli Oil (Citrus aurantium), 100ml distilled water, 1 tsp Witch Hazel, Spray bottle

Process: Brew a strong green tea and let it cool. Mix the tea with Witch Hazel, Green Tea Extract, and Neroli Oil in a spray bottle. Shake well. Use as a refreshing facial mist throughout the day.

Revitalizing Coffee Eye Cream

P.T.: 12 minutes

Ingr.: 2 tsp Coffee Oil (infused from ground coffee beans), 3 drops Vitamin E Oil, 20g Cocoa Butter (Theobroma cacao), 10ml Coconut Oil (Cocos nucifera), Small container

Process: Gently melt Cocoa Butter and Coconut Oil in a double boiler. Remove from heat and add Coffee and Vitamin E oils. Pour into a container and let it solidify. Apply under the eyes to reduce puffiness and dark circles.

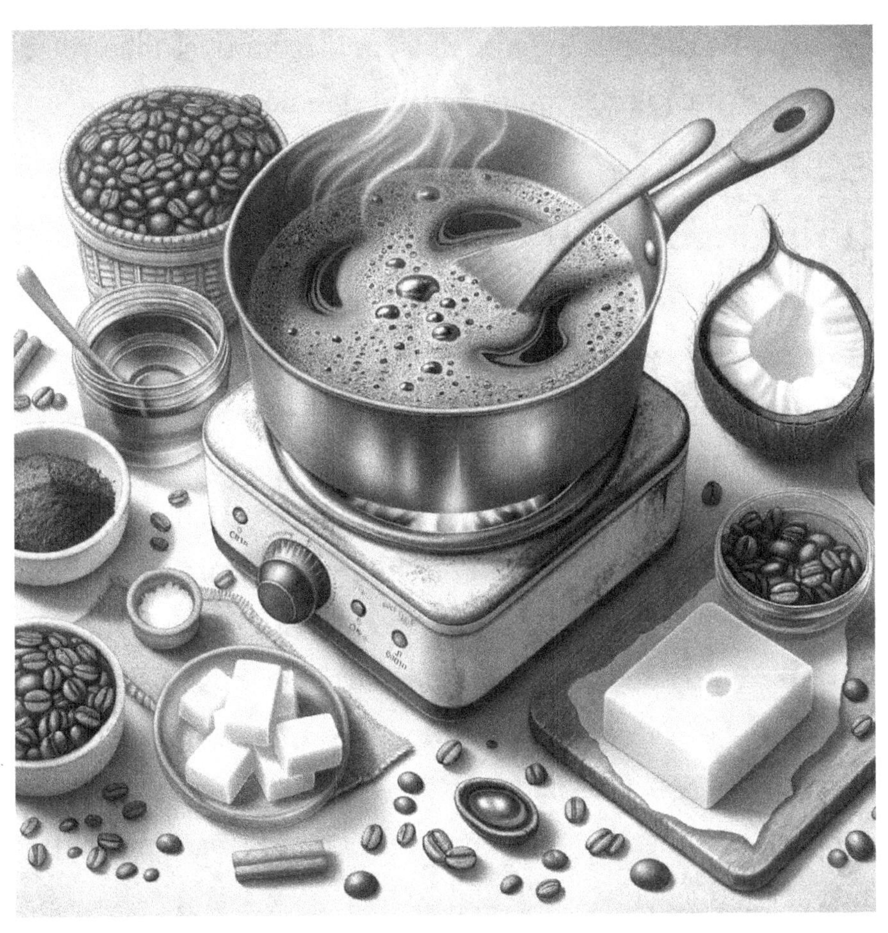

Gentle Oatmeal Exfoliating Scrub

P.T.: 10 minutes

Ingr.: 4 drops Geranium Oil (Pelargonium graveolens), 1/2 cup Ground Oatmeal, 1/4 cup Honey, 2 tbsp Olive Oil (Olea europaea), Mixing bowl

Process: In a bowl, combine Ground Oatmeal, Honey, and Olive Oil. Add Geranium Oil and mix until a paste forms.

Gently massage onto the face in a circular motion, then rinse. Use weekly for gentle exfoliation and skin nourishment.

Hair Care Elixirs and Treatments

Revitalizing Rosemary Scalp Serum

P.T.: 10 minutes

Ingr.: 5 drops Rosemary Oil (Rosmarinus officinalis), 4 drops Lavender Oil (Lavandula angustifolia), 30ml Jojoba Oil (Simmondsia chinensis), 20ml Castor Oil (Ricinus communis)

Process: Combine Rosemary and Lavender oils with Jojoba and Castor oils in a small bottle. Shake well to mix. Massage into the scalp before bedtime to stimulate hair growth and improve scalp health. Leave on overnight and wash out in the morning.

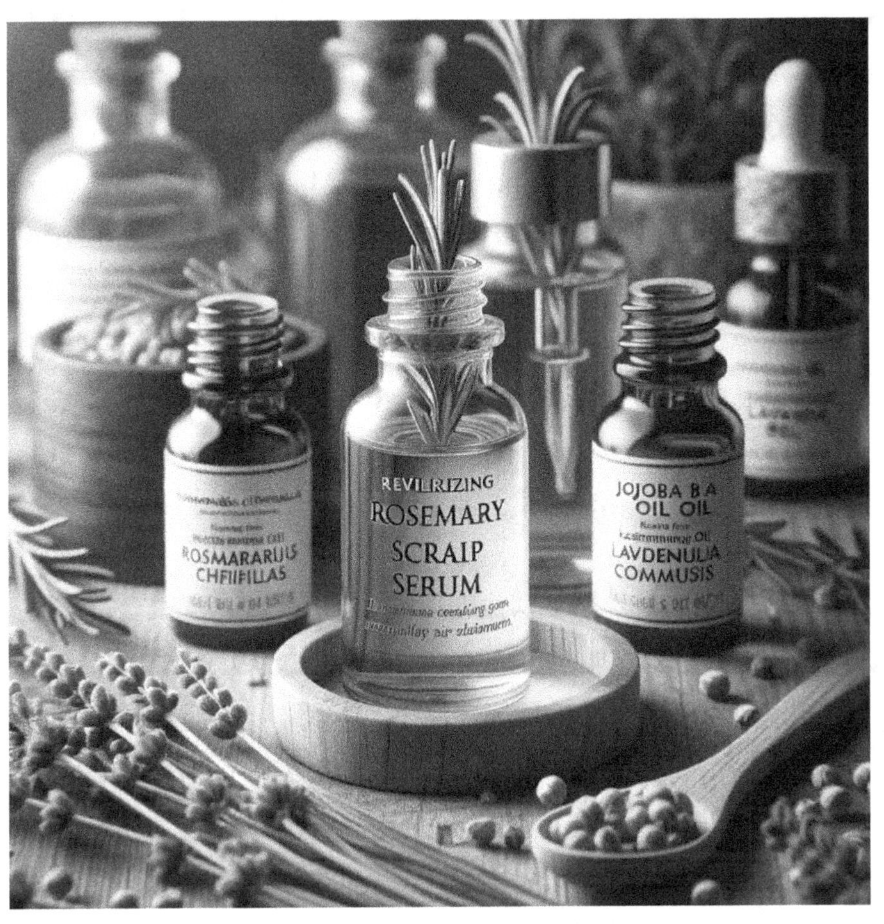

Hydrating Avocado Hair Mask

P.T.: 15 minutes

Ingr.: 1 ripe Avocado, 3 drops Ylang Ylang Oil (Cananga odorata), 2 tbsp Olive Oil (Olea europaea), 1 tbsp Honey

Process: Mash the Avocado in a bowl. Add Ylang Ylang Oil, Olive Oil, and Honey. Mix until smooth. Apply to hair, focusing on ends. Leave for 30 minutes, then rinse thoroughly.

Strengthening Protein Hair Treatment

P.T.: 20 minutes

Ingr.: 1 Egg, 4 drops Peppermint Oil (Mentha piperita), 50ml Coconut Milk (Cocos nucifera), 2 tbsp Coconut Oil (Cocos nucifera)

Process: Whisk the Egg in a bowl. Add Peppermint Oil, Coconut Milk, and Coconut Oil. Apply the mixture to your hair, cover with a shower cap, and leave for 20-30 minutes. Rinse with cool water and shampoo.

Clarifying Apple Cider Vinegar Rinse

P.T.: 5 minutes

Ingr.: 100ml Apple Cider Vinegar (Malus domestica), 3 drops Tea Tree Oil (Melaleuca alternifolia), 400ml Water

Process: Mix Apple Cider Vinegar, Tea Tree Oil, and Water in a large bottle. After shampooing, apply the rinse to your hair, ensuring full coverage. Leave for 2-3 minutes, then rinse with cool water.

Nourishing Argan Leave-In Conditioner

P.T.: 10 minutes

Ingr.: 5 drops Argan Oil (Argania spinosa), 3 drops Sandalwood Oil (Santalum album), 50ml Aloe Vera Gel (Aloe barbadensis), 50ml Distilled Water

Process: In a spray bottle, combine Argan Oil, Sandalwood Oil, Aloe Vera Gel, and Distilled Water. Shake well to blend. Spray onto damp hair after washing as a leave-in conditioner to moisturize and add shine.

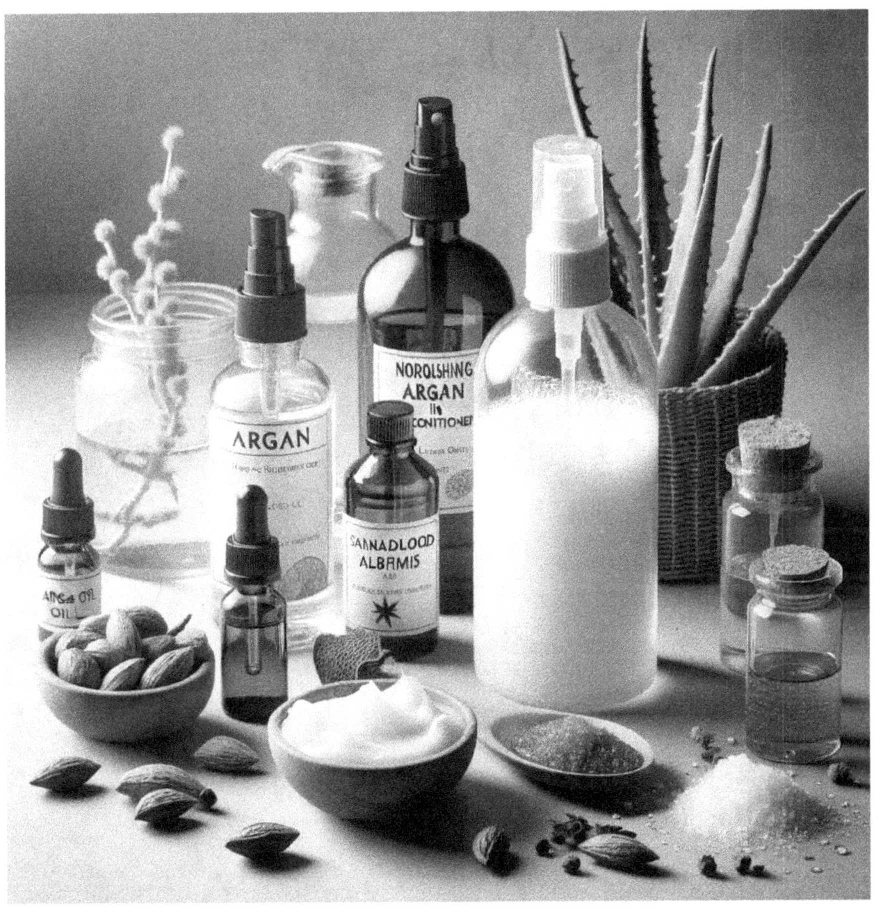

Natural Oral Care Blends

<table><tr><td><h2 align="center">Minty Fresh Mouthwash</h2></td></tr></table>

P.T.: 10 minutes

Ingr.: 5 drops Peppermint Oil (Mentha piperita), 3 drops Tea Tree Oil (Melaleuca alternifolia), 250ml Distilled Water, 1 tbsp Witch Hazel (Hamamelis virginiana)

Process: In a bottle, combine Peppermint and Tea Tree oils with Witch Hazel. Add Distilled Water and shake well. Use as a mouthwash daily for fresh breath and antibacterial benefits.

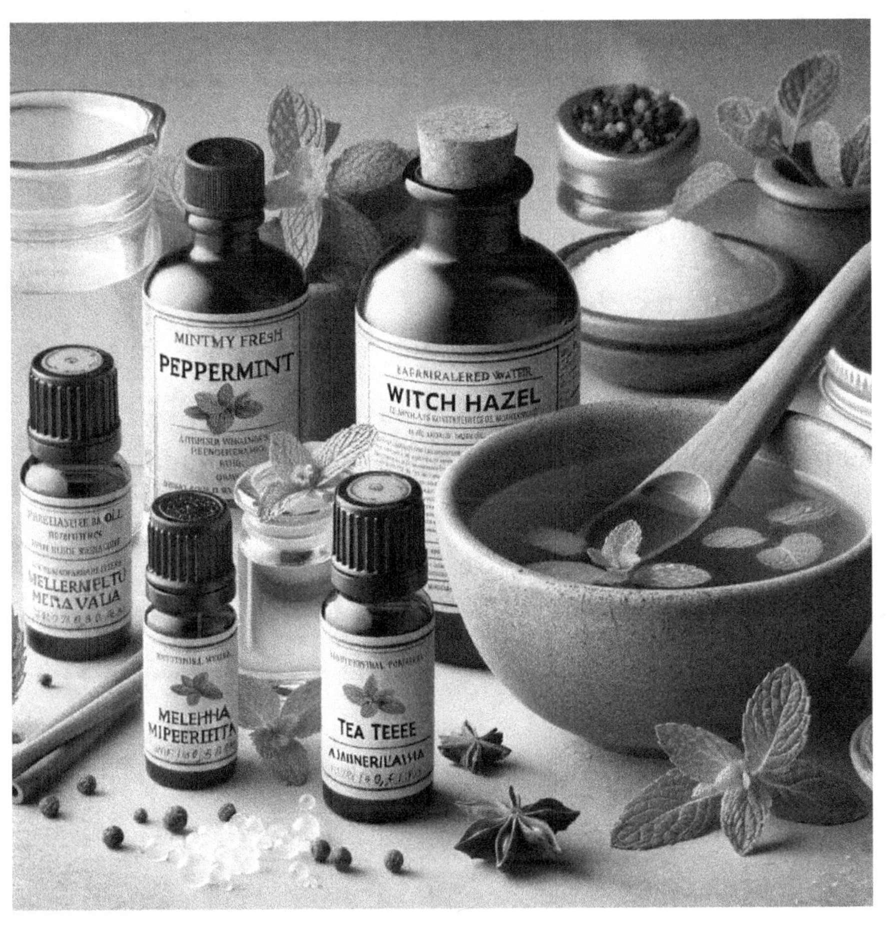

Cinnamon Clove Toothpaste

P.T.: 15 minutes

Ingr.: 2 drops Cinnamon Oil (Cinnamomum zeylanicum), 2 drops Clove Oil (Eugenia caryophyllata), 3 tbsp Baking Soda (Sodium bicarbonate), 2 tbsp Coconut Oil (Cocos nucifera)

Process: Mix Baking Soda with melted Coconut Oil. Add Cinnamon and Clove oils. Store in a small jar and use as toothpaste for its antibacterial and refreshing properties.

Herbal Gum Serum

P.T.: 10 minutes

Ingr.: 4 drops Myrrh Oil (Commiphora myrrha), 3 drops Frankincense Oil (Boswellia carterii), 30ml Fractionated Coconut Oil (Cocos nucifera)

Process: Combine Myrrh and Frankincense oils with Fractionated Coconut Oil in a dropper bottle. Apply a drop to gums and massage gently to reduce inflammation and promote gum health.

Lemon Whitening Rinse

P.T.: 5 minutes

Ingr.: 4 drops Lemon Oil (Citrus limon), 250ml Distilled Water, 1 tsp Baking Soda (Sodium bicarbonate)

Process: Dissolve Baking Soda in Distilled Water. Add Lemon Oil and mix well. Use as a mouth rinse to naturally whiten teeth and remove stains.

Soothing Aloe Vera Mouth Gel

P.T.: 10 minutes

Ingr.: 3 drops Spearmint Oil (Mentha spicata), 2 drops Lavender Oil (Lavandula angustifolia), 50ml Aloe Vera Gel (Aloe barbadensis)

Process: Mix Spearmint and Lavender oils with Aloe Vera Gel. Store in a small container. Apply to mouth ulcers or sore gums for soothing relief.

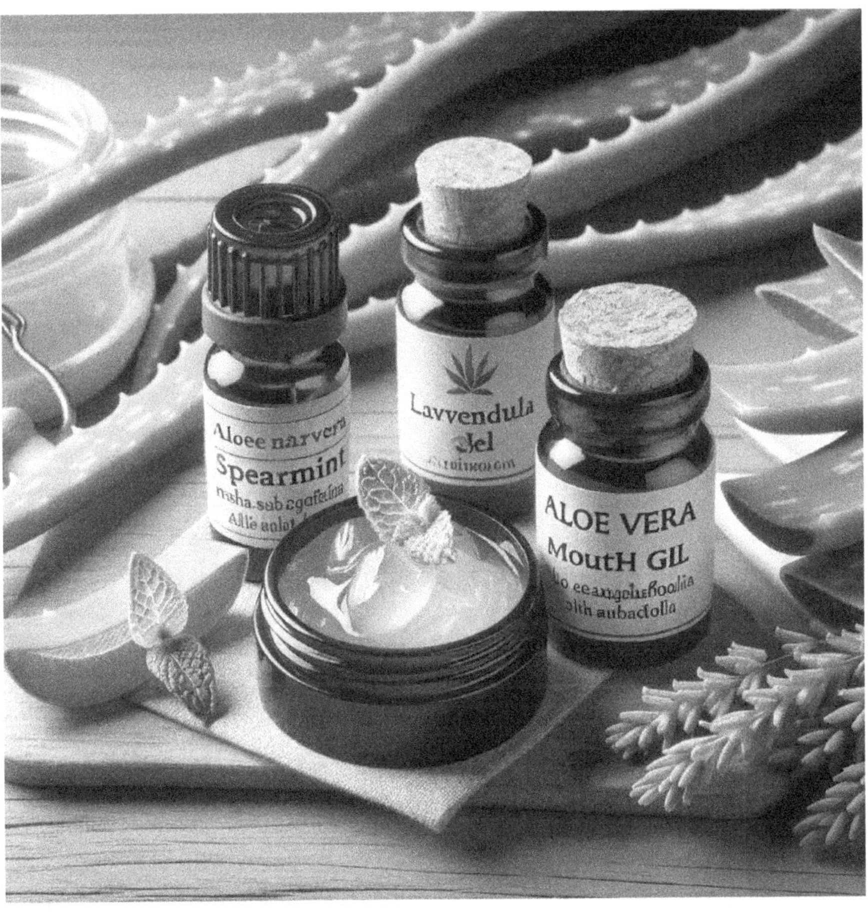

As we wrap up our exploration of personal care potions, we reflect on the enriching experience of integrating natural, essential oil-based products into our self-care rituals. This chapter has been a journey through a variety of recipes, each showcasing the diverse and powerful roles of essential oils in personal care. From skin nourishment to hair revitalization, and maintaining oral hygiene, these natural concoctions have demonstrated their significant impact on our health and wellness. Adopting these recipes into our daily lives not only offers practical benefits but also deepens our connection with the natural world, fostering a mindful and holistic approach to self-care. By choosing these natural potions, we commit to a lifestyle that values sustainability and holistic health, celebrating the simplicity and profound benefits of natural wellness.

CHAPTER 2: Holistic Home Care

Embarking on a journey of Holistic Home Care, this chapter introduces a world where the purity and efficacy of natural ingredients take center stage in maintaining a clean, healthy, and harmonious living space. We delve into the art of creating eco-friendly cleaning solutions, air freshening blends, and natural pest repellents, all crafted with essential oils and safe, non-toxic ingredients. These recipes not only aim to keep homes clean and fresh but also ensure a living environment that nurtures well-being and respects the earth. The focus here is on harnessing the power of nature's essences to create effective home care solutions that are kind to both our health and the planet. Through these pages, we invite you to transform everyday cleaning and home maintenance into a practice of mindful living and environmental stewardship.

Eco-Friendly Cleaning Solutions

Citrus Burst All-Purpose Cleaner

P.T.: 10 minutes

Ingr.: 5 drops Lemon Oil (Citrus limon), 5 drops Orange Oil (Citrus sinensis), 250ml White Vinegar, 250ml Water, Spray bottle

Process: Combine Lemon and Orange oils with White Vinegar and Water in a spray bottle. Shake well to mix. Use this solution to clean surfaces, kitchens, and bathrooms for a natural, citrus-fresh clean.

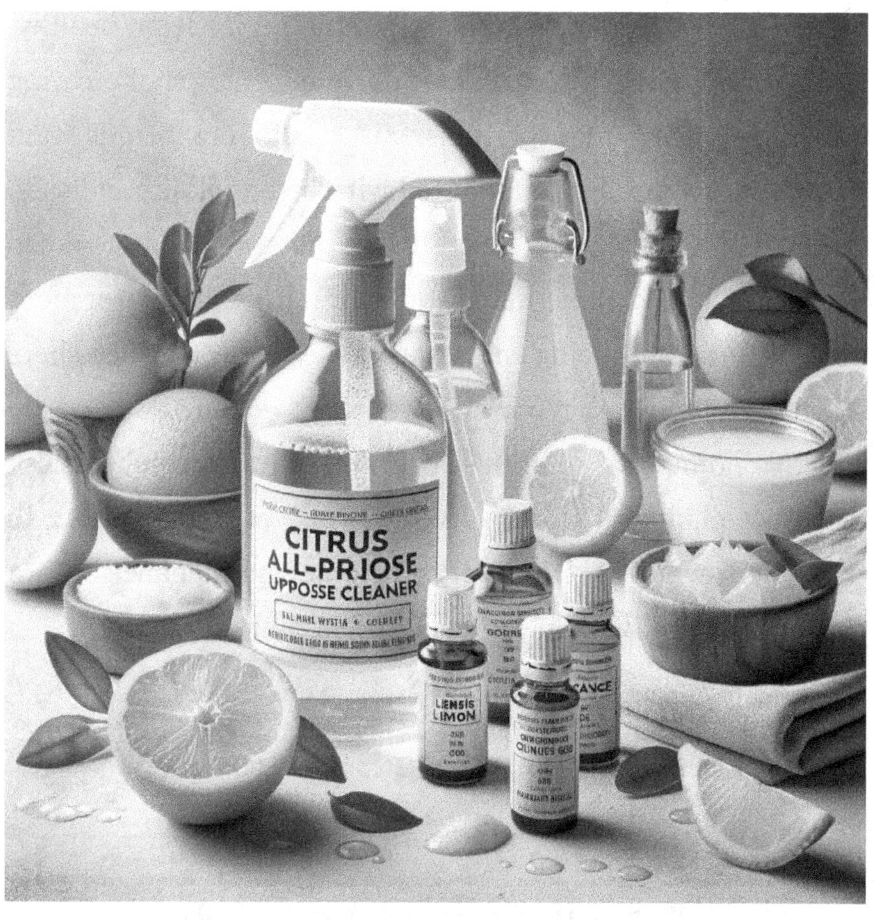

Herbal Floor Freshener

P.T.: 8 minutes

Ingr.: 4 drops Lavender Oil (Lavandula angustifolia), 4 drops Rosemary Oil (Rosmarinus officinalis), 500ml Hot Water, 100ml White Vinegar

Process: Mix Lavender and Rosemary oils with Hot Water and White Vinegar in a bucket. Use this blend to mop floors for a naturally clean and aromatic finish.

Sparkling Window Wash

P.T.: 5 minutes

Ingr.: 6 drops Peppermint Oil (Mentha piperita), 250ml White Vinegar, 250ml Water, Spray bottle

Process: Combine Peppermint Oil with White Vinegar and Water in a spray bottle. Use this minty mixture to clean windows and glass surfaces, leaving a streak-free shine.

Grease Fighter Kitchen Scrub

P.T.: 7 minutes

Ingr.: 3 drops Lemon Oil (Citrus limon), 3 drops Eucalyptus Oil (Eucalyptus globulus), 2 tbsp Baking Soda, 1 tbsp Liquid Castile Soap

Process: Blend Lemon and Eucalyptus oils with Baking Soda and Liquid Castile Soap to form a paste. Apply this scrub to kitchen surfaces to tackle tough grease and grime effectively.

Mold and Mildew Remover

P.T.: 6 minutes

Ingr.: 5 drops Tea Tree Oil (Melaleuca alternifolia), 250ml Water, 250ml White Vinegar, Spray bottle

Process: Mix Tea Tree Oil with Water and White Vinegar in a spray bottle. Spray on areas prone to mold and mildew. Leave for a few minutes before scrubbing off. This solution works well in damp areas like bathrooms.

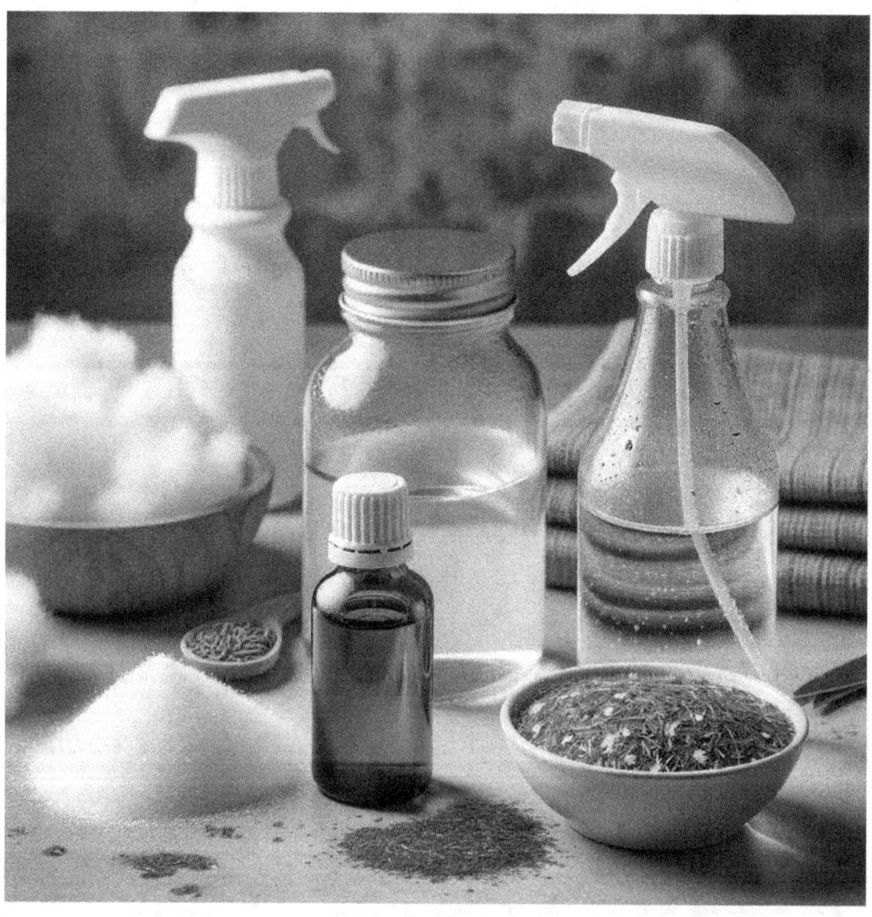

Air Freshening and Purification Blends

Refreshing Citrus Grove Diffuser Blend

P.T.: 3 minutes

Ingr.: 4 drops Grapefruit Oil (Citrus paradisi), 3 drops Lemon Oil (Citrus limon), 2 drops Bergamot Oil (Citrus bergamia), Diffuser

Process: Add Grapefruit, Lemon, and Bergamot oils to a diffuser filled with water. Use this blend to create a refreshing and uplifting atmosphere, reminiscent of a citrus grove.

Forest Freshness Room Spray

P.T.: 5 minutes

Ingr.: 5 drops Pine Oil (Pinus sylvestris), 4 drops Cedarwood Oil (Cedrus atlantica), 100ml Distilled Water, 1 tsp Witch Hazel, Spray bottle

Process: Mix Pine and Cedarwood oils with Witch Hazel in a spray bottle. Add Distilled Water and shake well. Spray around the room for a forest-like freshness and natural air purification.

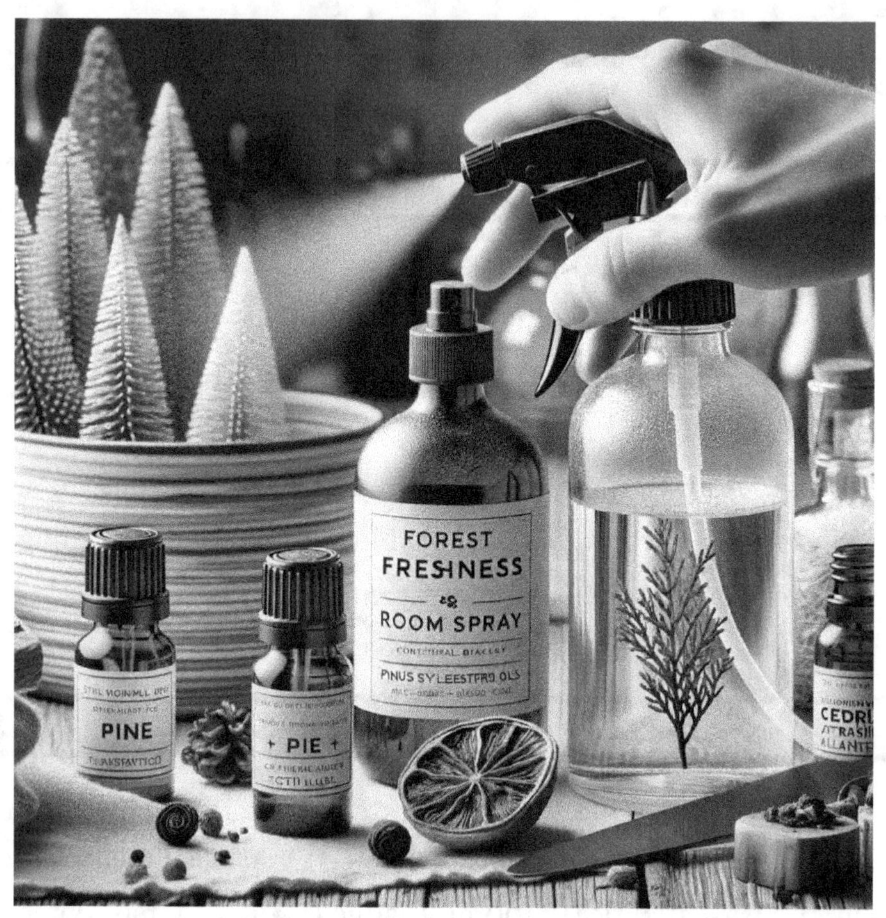

Soothing Lavender Vanilla Mist

P.T.: 4 minutes

Ingr.: 5 drops Lavender Oil (Lavandula angustifolia), 2 drops Vanilla Extract, 100ml Distilled Water, 1 tsp Witch Hazel, Spray bottle

Process: Blend Lavender Oil and Vanilla Extract with Witch Hazel in a spray bottle. Add Distilled Water and shake well.

Use as a calming room spray, ideal for bedrooms or relaxation spaces.

Energizing Peppermint Eucalyptus Diffusion

P.T.: 2 minutes

Ingr.: 4 drops Peppermint Oil (Mentha piperita), 4 drops Eucalyptus Oil (Eucalyptus globulus), Diffuser

Process: Combine Peppermint and Eucalyptus oils in a diffuser with water. This blend is perfect for energizing a room while purifying the air.

Herbal Harmony Aroma Blend

P.T.: 3 minutes

Ingr.: 3 drops Rosemary Oil (Rosmarinus officinalis), 3 drops Thyme Oil (Thymus vulgaris), 2 drops Lemon Oil (Citrus limon), Diffuser

Process: Add Rosemary, Thyme, and Lemon oils to a diffuser filled with water. Use this aromatic blend to create a harmonious and clean-smelling environment, perfect for kitchens or living spaces.

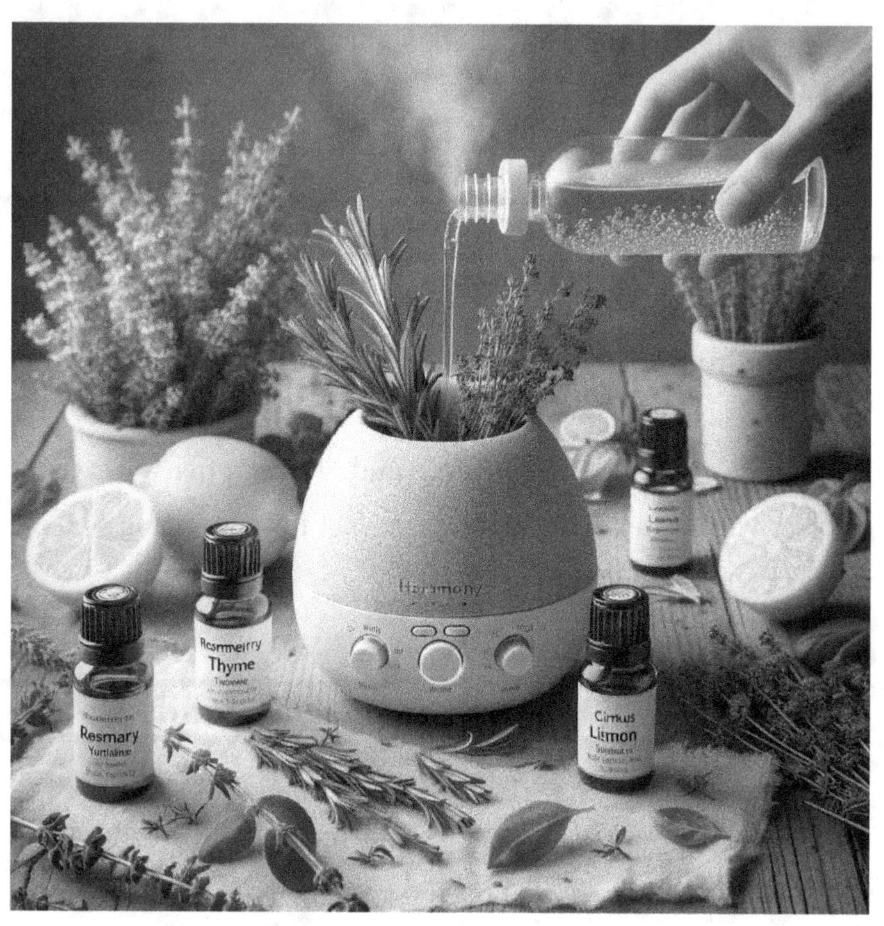

Natural Pest Repellents

Lemongrass Ant Repellent Spray

P.T.: 5 minutes

Ingr.: 10 drops Lemongrass Oil (Cymbopogon citratus), 250ml
Water, 1 tbsp Dish Soap, Spray bottle

Process: Mix Lemongrass Oil with Water and Dish Soap in a spray bottle. Shake well. Spray around doorways, windowsills, and areas where ants are present.

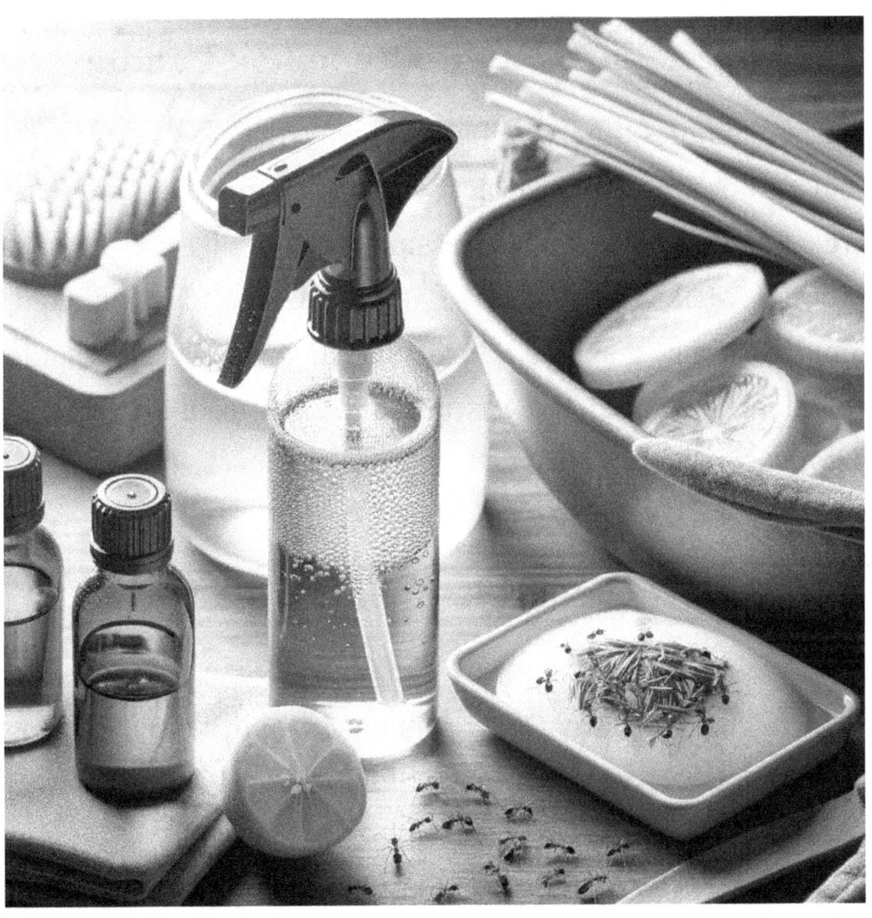

Peppermint Rodent Deterrent

P.T.: 3 minutes

Ingr.: 12 drops Peppermint Oil (Mentha piperita), 250ml Water, Spray bottle

Process: Combine Peppermint Oil with Water in a spray bottle. Spray in corners, cupboards, and potential rodent entry points. Reapply every few days or as needed.

Citronella Mosquito Repellent Candle

P.T.: 20 minutes (plus cooling time)

Ingr.: 30 drops Citronella Oil (Cymbopogon nardus), 500g Soy Wax, Candle wicks, Candle containers

Process: Melt Soy Wax in a double boiler. Once melted, remove from heat and add Citronella Oil. Place wicks in candle containers and pour the wax mixture. Let it cool and solidify before use.

Clove Tick Repellant Blend

P.T.: 5 minutes

Ingr.: 8 drops Clove Oil (Eugenia caryophyllata), 6 drops Lavender Oil (Lavandula angustifolia), 30ml Grapeseed Oil, Small container

Process: Mix Clove and Lavender oils with Grapeseed Oil in a small container. Apply to skin before going outdoors to repel ticks.

Eucalyptus Spider Repellent Spray

P.T.: 4 minutes

Ingr.: 10 drops Eucalyptus Oil (Eucalyptus globulus), 250ml
Water, 1 tbsp White Vinegar, Spray bottle
Process: Blend Eucalyptus Oil with Water and White Vinegar
in a spray bottle. Spray in corners, closets, and areas where
spiders are frequently seen.

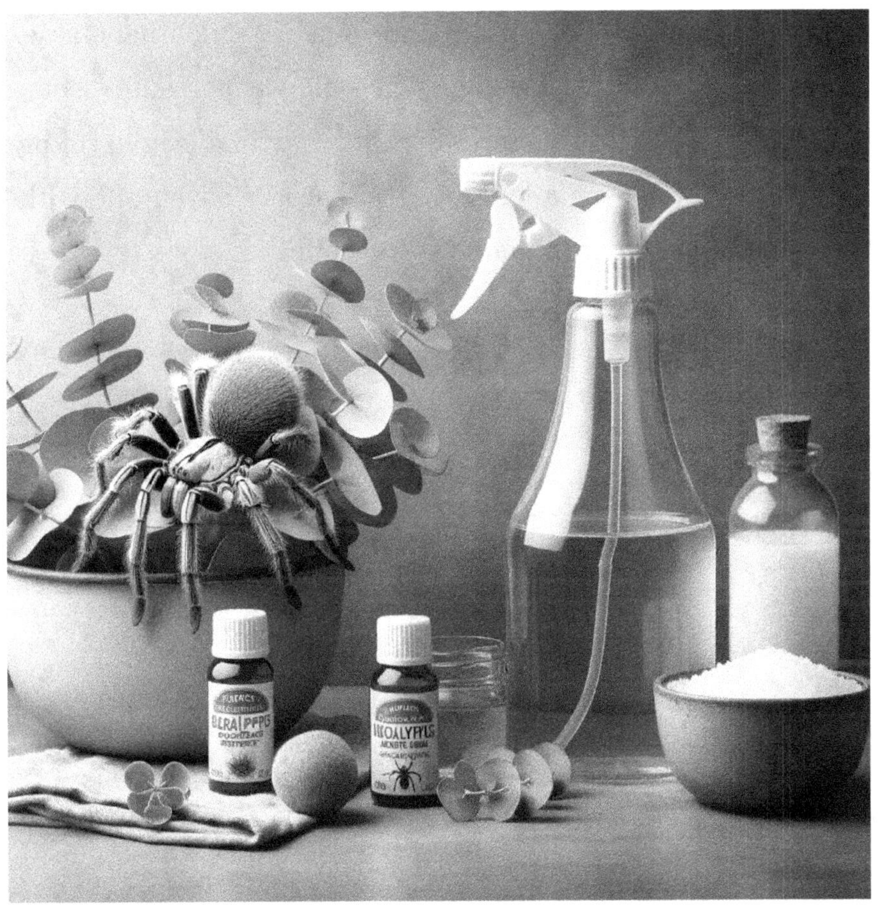

As we conclude our exploration of Holistic Home Care, we are
equipped with a collection of natural recipes and solutions that

redefine the essence of home maintenance. This chapter has been a testament to the power of nature in creating a home environment that is not only clean and refreshing but also health-conscious and eco-friendly. From the invigorating scents of homemade cleaning agents to the gentle efficacy of air purifiers and the strategic repelling of pests, these natural solutions embody a commitment to a lifestyle that values sustainability and well-being. The knowledge gained here empowers us to care for our homes in a way that is in harmony with nature, fostering a living space that is a haven of health, tranquility, and environmental responsibility.

CHAPTER 3: Nutritional Enhancements

Embarking on a culinary adventure, this chapter unfolds the innovative use of essential oils in enhancing the nutritional and sensory aspects of food and beverages. We explore the art of incorporating these potent essences into our daily diet, from flavoring foods to enriching beverages and harnessing their preservative qualities. Each recipe and application presents a unique way to infuse natural flavors and health benefits into everyday meals and drinks. This exploration is not just about adding aroma and taste; it's a journey towards understanding the subtle yet significant impact of essential oils on our overall well-being. Through these pages, we invite you to transform your culinary practices with the essence of nature, blending tradition with modern insights for a holistic approach to nutrition.

Flavoring Food with Essential Oils

Lemon Herb Roasted Chicken

P.T.: 1 hour 20 minutes

Ingr.: 1 whole chicken, 2 drops Lemon Oil (Citrus limon), 1 tbsp olive oil, 1 tsp sea salt, 1/2 tsp black pepper, 2 sprigs fresh rosemary, 2 sprigs fresh thyme

Process: Preheat oven to 375°F (190°C). Mix Lemon Oil with olive oil, salt, and pepper. Rub the mixture all over the chicken. Place rosemary and thyme inside the chicken cavity. Roast for 1 hour or until the chicken is cooked through.

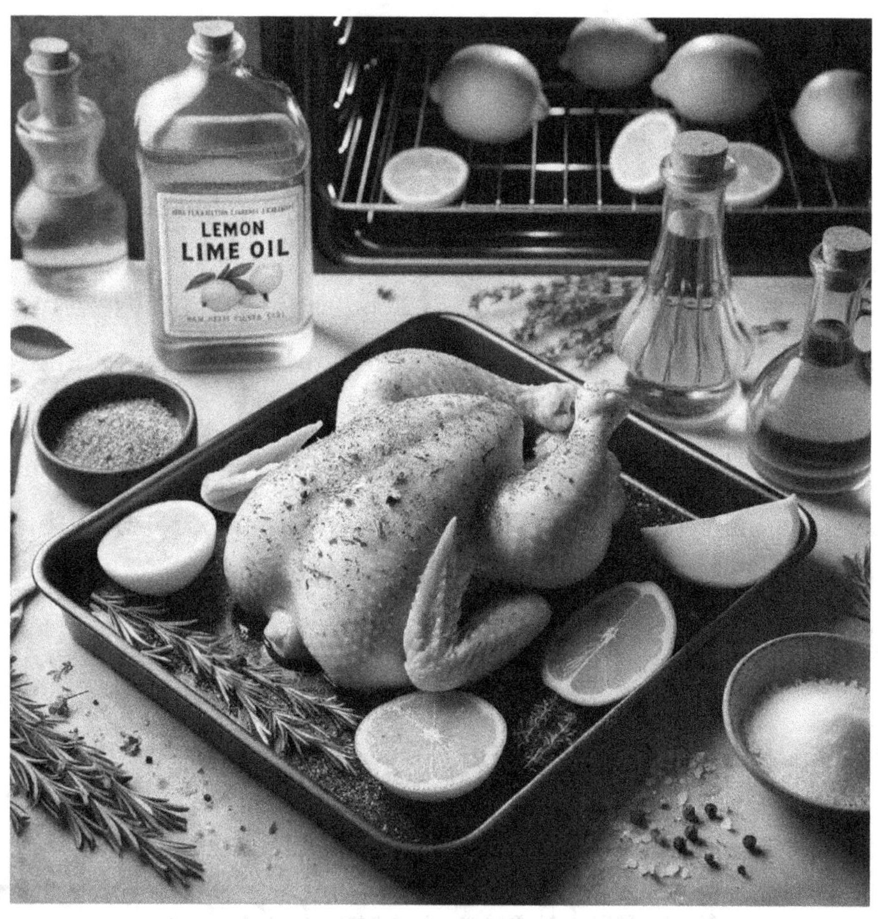

Peppermint Chocolate Brownies

P.T.: 35 minutes

Ingr.: 2 cups all-purpose flour, 1 cup unsweetened cocoa powder, 1 1/2 cups sugar, 1/2 cup melted butter, 2 eggs, 1 drop Peppermint Oil (Mentha piperita), 1/4 tsp salt

Process: Preheat oven to 350°F (175°C). Mix all dry ingredients. Add eggs, butter, and Peppermint Oil; stir until well combined. Pour batter into a greased baking pan. Bake for 20-25 minutes.

Citrus Infused Salad Dressing

P.T.: 10 minutes

Ingr.: 1 drop Orange Oil (Citrus sinensis), 1 drop Lemon Oil (Citrus limon), 1/4 cup olive oil, 2 tbsp apple cider vinegar, 1 tsp honey, Salt and pepper to taste

Process: Whisk together Orange and Lemon oils, olive oil, vinegar, and honey. Season with salt and pepper. Toss with your favorite salad.

Rosemary Garlic Mashed Potatoes

P.T.: 30 minutes

Ingr.: 4 large potatoes, peeled and quartered, 1 drop Rosemary Oil (Rosmarinus officinalis), 2 cloves garlic, minced, 1/4 cup milk, 2 tbsp butter, Salt to taste

Process: Boil potatoes until tender. Mash with garlic, milk, butter, Rosemary Oil, and salt.

Basil Oil Infused Pasta

P.T.: 20 minutes

Ingr.: 1 drop Basil Oil (Ocimum basilicum), 12 oz. pasta, 1/4 cup grated Parmesan cheese, 1/4 cup olive oil, 1/2 cup cherry tomatoes, halved, Salt and pepper to taste

Process: Cook pasta according to package instructions. Drain and return to pot. Stir in olive oil, Basil Oil, Parmesan, tomatoes, salt, and pepper. Serve warm.

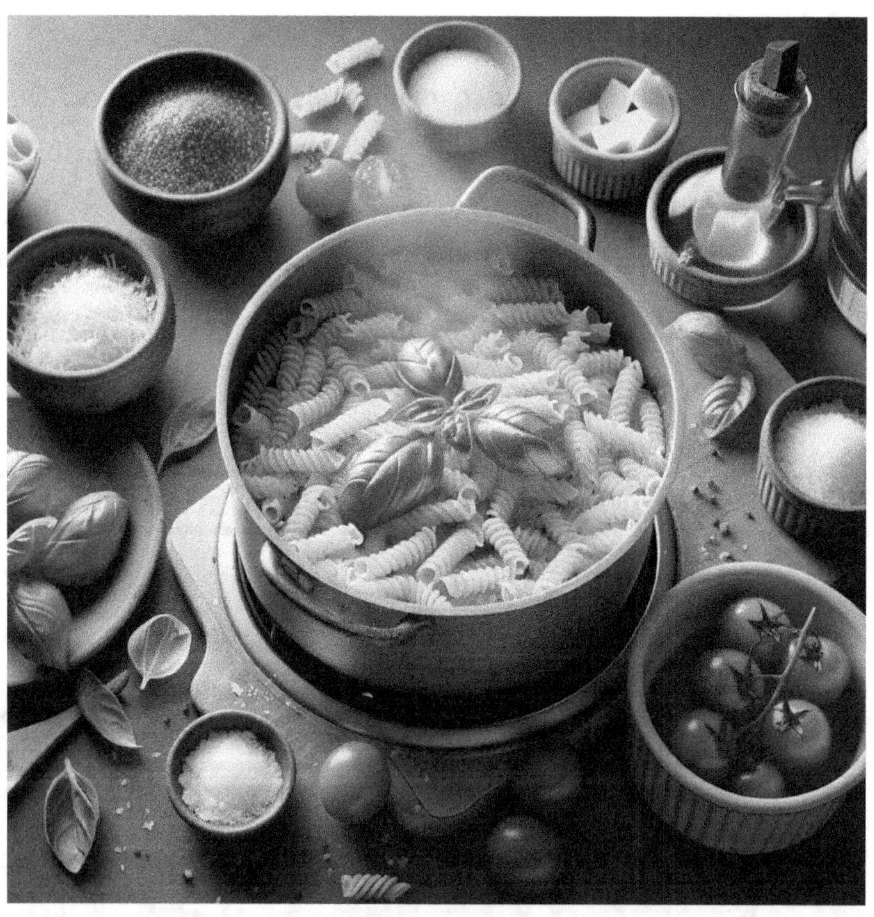

Essential Oils in Beverages and Cocktails

Minty Citrus Cooler

P.T.: 5 minutes

Ingr.: 2 drops Peppermint Oil (Mentha piperita), 1 drop Lemon Oil (Citrus limon), 1 tbsp honey, Juice of 2 oranges, Sparkling water, Ice cubes

Process: In a glass, dissolve honey with a small amount of hot water. Add Peppermint and Lemon oils, orange juice, and stir. Fill the glass with ice cubes, top with sparkling water, and stir gently.

Lavender Lemonade

P.T.: 10 minutes

Ingr.: 1 drop Lavender Oil (Lavandula angustifolia), Juice of 4 lemons, 4 cups water, 1/2 cup sugar or honey

Process: In a pitcher, dissolve sugar or honey in 1 cup of warm water. Add Lavender Oil, lemon juice, and remaining water. Chill in the refrigerator. Serve over ice.

Ginger Spice Tea

P.T.: 15 minutes

Ingr.: 1 drop Ginger Oil (Zingiber officinale), 1 black tea bag, 1 tsp honey, 1 cup boiling water, Lemon slice

Process: Steep tea bag in boiling water for 5 minutes. Remove the tea bag, add Ginger Oil and honey. Stir well. Serve with a lemon slice.

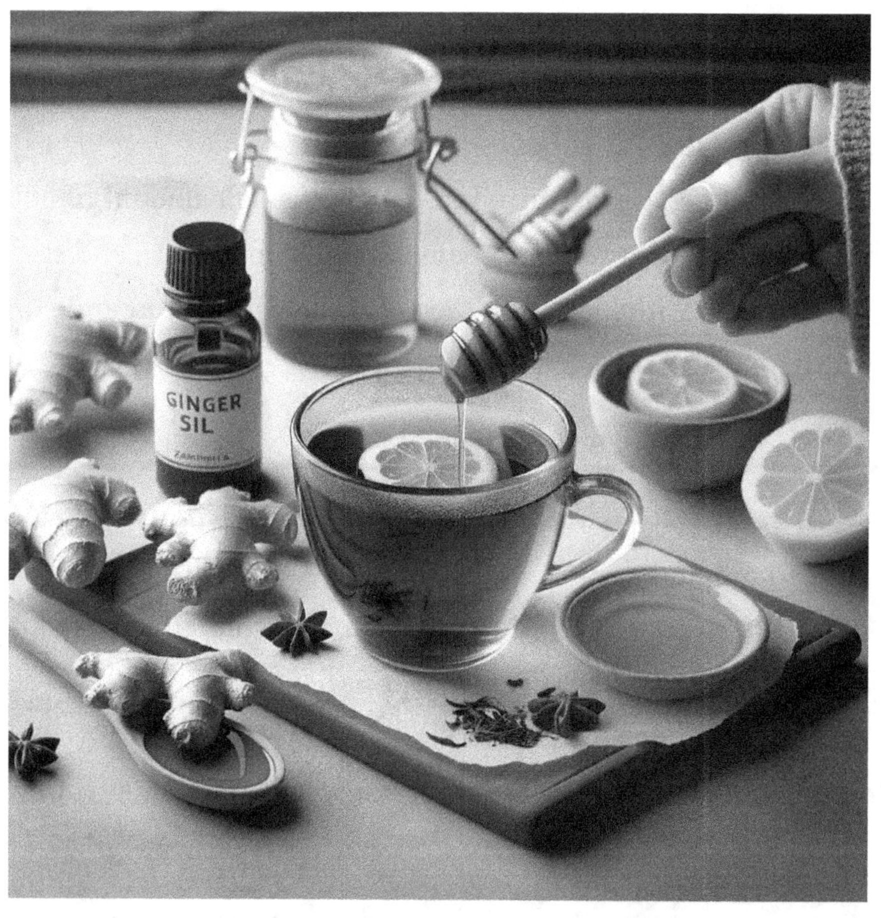

Herbal Mojito Mocktail

P.T.: 5 minutes

Ingr.: 2 drops Spearmint Oil (Mentha spicata), Juice of 1 lime, 1 tsp sugar, Sparkling water, Fresh mint leaves, Ice cubes

Process: Muddle mint leaves with sugar and lime juice in a glass. Add Spearmint Oil and stir. Fill the glass with ice cubes, top with sparkling water, and mix gently.

Rosemary Citrus Spritz

P.T.: 7 minutes

Ingr.: 1 drop Rosemary Oil (Rosmarinus officinalis), Juice of 1 grapefruit, 1/2 cup orange juice, Sparkling water, Rosemary sprig for garnish, Ice cubes

Process: In a glass, combine grapefruit juice, orange juice, and Rosemary Oil. Fill the glass with ice cubes and top with sparkling water. Garnish with a sprig of rosemary.

Preservative Effects of Essential Oils

Citrus Oil Fruit Preserver

P.T.: 5 minutes

Ingr.: 2 drops Lemon Oil (Citrus limon), 2 drops Grapefruit Oil (Citrus paradisi), 1 liter Water

Process: Mix Lemon and Grapefruit oils in water. Soak freshly cut fruits in the solution for a few minutes to prevent browning and extend freshness. Drain and store the fruits in the refrigerator.

Herbal Bread Freshener

P.T.: 10 minutes

Ingr.: 1 drop Rosemary Oil (Rosmarinus officinalis), 1 drop Thyme Oil (Thymus vulgaris), 1 cup Warm Water, 1 tbsp Vinegar

Process: Blend Rosemary and Thyme oils with warm water and vinegar. Brush the solution lightly over bread before storing to prevent mold and keep it fresh longer.

Natural Meat Marinade Preserver

P.T.: 15 minutes

Ingr.: 2 drops Oregano Oil (Origanum vulgare), 2 drops Lemon Oil (Citrus limon), 1/4 cup Olive Oil, Salt, Pepper

Process: Mix Oregano and Lemon oils with olive oil, salt, and pepper. Use as a marinade for meat. The essential oils help preserve the meat and enhance flavor.

Vegetable Wash and Preserver

P.T.: 7 minutes

Ingr.: 3 drops Peppermint Oil (Mentha piperita), 2 drops Tea Tree Oil (Melaleuca alternifolia), 1 liter Water

Process: Combine Peppermint and Tea Tree oils with water. Soak vegetables in the mixture to clean and extend their shelf life. Rinse thoroughly before storage.

Antioxidant Spice Mix for Preserving Nuts

P.T.: 5 minutes

Ingr.: 2 drops Clove Oil (Eugenia caryophyllata), 1 drop Cinnamon Oil (Cinnamomum zeylanicum), 1/2 cup Raw Nuts, Pinch of Salt

Process: Blend Clove and Cinnamon oils with a pinch of salt. Toss nuts in the mixture and spread them on a baking sheet. Roast lightly to infuse the flavors and preserve freshness. Store in an airtight container.

As we conclude our exploration of nutritional enhancements with essential oils, we carry with us a deeper appreciation for the versatility and potency of these natural extracts in culinary applications. This chapter has been a journey through a variety of creative recipes and techniques, showcasing how essential oils can elevate the flavors, nutritional value, and preservation of our food and drinks. From the zesty twists in beverages to the aromatic depths in meals and the innovative preservation techniques, these natural essences have opened new dimensions in our culinary experiences. Incorporating these essential oil-infused recipes into our daily lives, we embrace a lifestyle that values natural wellness, flavor richness, and culinary innovation, all while maintaining a harmonious balance with nature's gifts.

CHAPTER 4: Therapeutic Blends

This chapter delves into the art and science of creating therapeutic blends, harnessing the potent benefits of essential oils to address common ailments, soothe the body, and support emotional well-being. It is a journey through the healing power of aromatherapy, where each blend is carefully crafted to provide relief, comfort, and balance. We explore remedies for everyday health concerns, from relieving headaches to aiding digestion, alongside soothing massage oil combinations that promote relaxation and muscle relief. The chapter also highlights synergistic blends designed to uplift, calm, and support the emotional spectrum, demonstrating the holistic approach of essential oils in nurturing both mind and body. This exploration is a testament to the versatility and effectiveness of essential oils, offering natural, holistic solutions for a variety of health and wellness needs.

Remedies for Common Ailments

Headache Relief Roll-On

P.T.: 5 minutes

Ingr.: 4 drops Peppermint Oil (Mentha piperita), 3 drops Lavender Oil (Lavandula angustifolia), 10ml Fractionated Coconut Oil (Cocos nucifera), Roll-on bottle

Process: Mix Peppermint and Lavender oils with Fractionated Coconut Oil in a roll-on bottle. Apply to temples, forehead, and back of the neck at the onset of a headache.

Digestive Comfort Massage Blend

P.T.: 5 minutes

Ingr.: 4 drops Ginger Oil (Zingiber officinale), 3 drops Fennel Oil (Foeniculum vulgare), 20ml Sweet Almond Oil (Prunus dulcis)

Process: Combine Ginger and Fennel oils with Sweet Almond Oil. Massage gently onto the abdomen in circular motions to ease digestive discomfort.

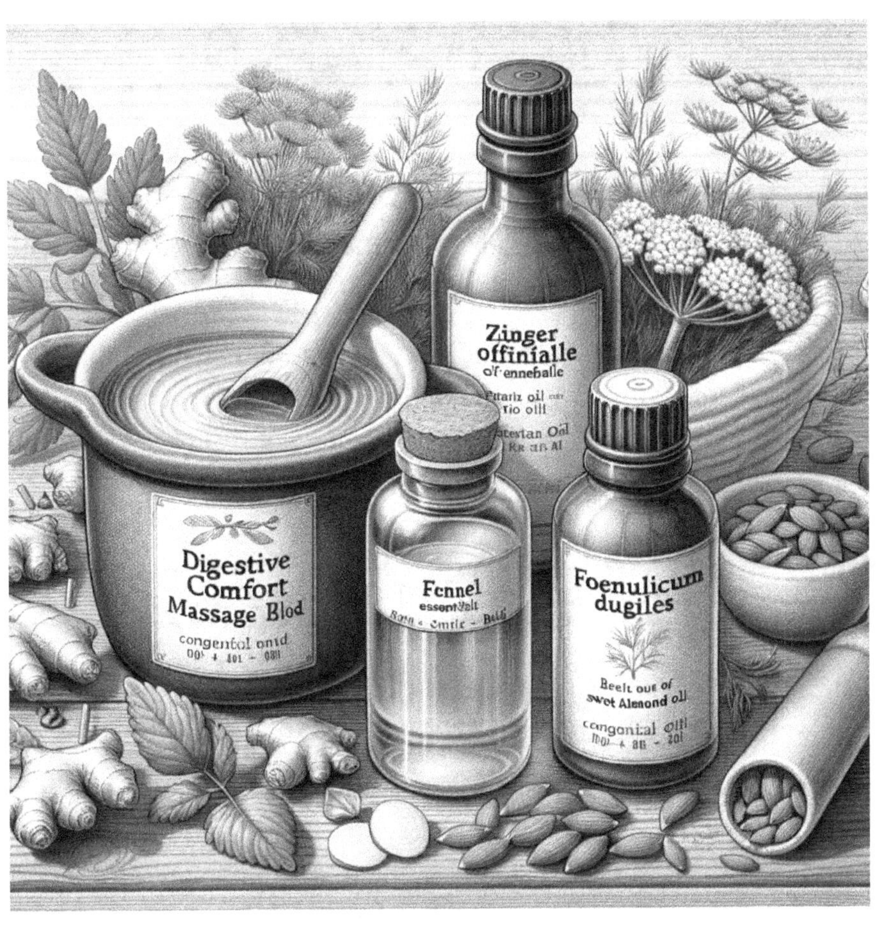

Cold and Flu Inhalation Blend

P.T.: 3 minutes

Ingr.: 3 drops Eucalyptus Oil (Eucalyptus globulus), 2 drops Tea Tree Oil (Melaleuca alternifolia), 1 drop Lemon Oil (Citrus limon), Bowl of hot water

Process: Add Eucalyptus, Tea Tree, and Lemon oils to a bowl of hot water. Inhale the steam to help clear congestion and soothe cold symptoms.

Muscle Soothe Massage Oil

P.T.: 6 minutes

Ingr.: 5 drops Marjoram Oil (Origanum majorana), 4 drops Rosemary Oil (Rosmarinus officinalis), 30ml Jojoba Oil (Simmondsia chinensis)

Process: Blend Marjoram and Rosemary oils with Jojoba Oil. Massage into sore muscles and joints for relief from aches and pains.

Sleep Enhancing Pillow Mist

P.T.: 5 minutes

Ingr.: 5 drops Lavender Oil (Lavandula angustifolia), 3 drops Chamomile Oil (Matricaria chamomilla), 100ml Distilled Water, Spray bottle

Process: Mix Lavender and Chamomile oils with Distilled Water in a spray bottle. Mist over pillows and bed linens before sleep to promote relaxation and better sleep quality.

Soothing Massage Oil Combinations

Relaxing Lavender Bliss Massage Oil

P.T.: 5 minutes

Ingr.: 5 drops Lavender Oil (Lavandula angustifolia), 3 drops Ylang Ylang Oil (Cananga odorata), 30ml Sweet Almond Oil (Prunus dulcis)

Process: Mix Lavender and Ylang Ylang oils with Sweet Almond Oil in a bottle. Shake well to blend. Use for a full-body massage to induce relaxation and reduce stress.

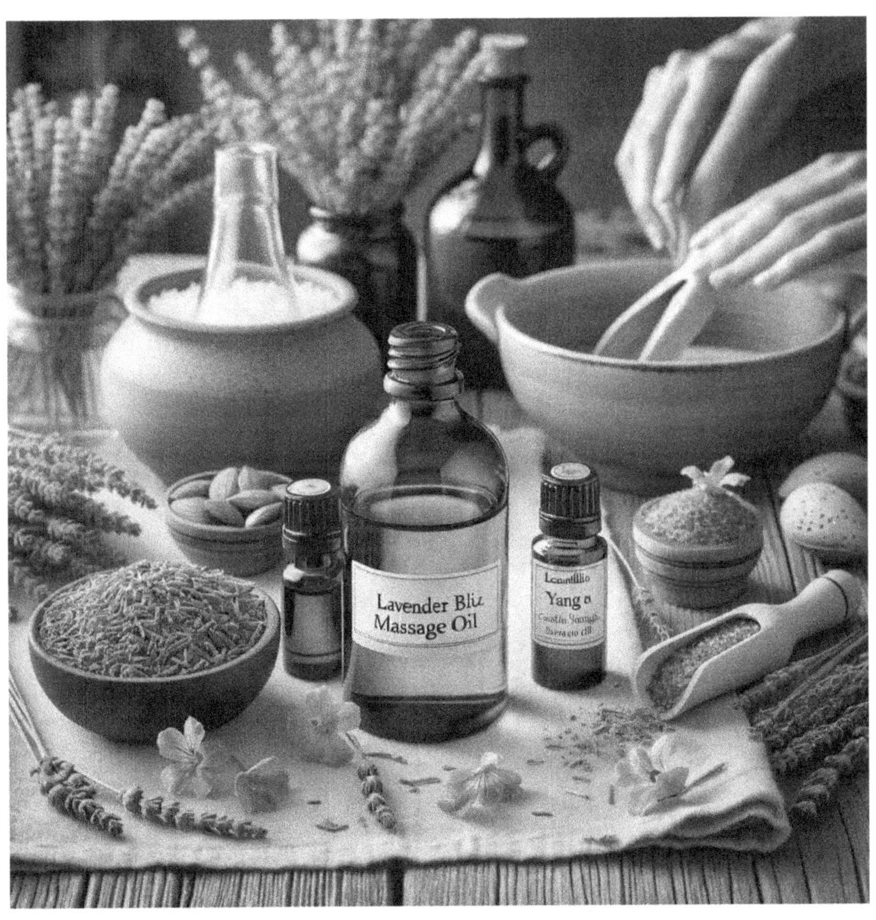

Energizing Citrus Boost Massage Oil

P.T.: 5 minutes

Ingr.: 4 drops Orange Oil (Citrus sinensis), 3 drops Grapefruit Oil (Citrus paradisi), 30ml Grapeseed Oil (Vitis vinifera)

Process: Combine Orange and Grapefruit oils with Grapeseed Oil in a bottle. Shake to mix thoroughly. Apply during massage to invigorate and uplift the mood.

Deep Muscle Relief Massage Oil

P.T.: 6 minutes

Ingr.: 5 drops Peppermint Oil (Mentha piperita), 4 drops Eucalyptus Oil (Eucalyptus globulus), 30ml Jojoba Oil (Simmondsia chinensis)

Process: Blend Peppermint and Eucalyptus oils with Jojoba Oil. Use for massaging sore and tired muscles for deep relief and a cooling sensation.

Calming Rosewood Serenity Massage Oil

P.T.: 5 minutes

Ingr.: 4 drops Rosewood Oil (Aniba rosaeodora), 3 drops Frankincense Oil (Boswellia carterii), 30ml Coconut Oil (Cocos nucifera)

Process: Mix Rosewood and Frankincense oils with Coconut Oil. This blend is ideal for a soothing massage that calms the mind and nurtures the skin.

Balancing Herbal Harmony Massage Oil

P.T.: 5 minutes

Ingr.: 3 drops Geranium Oil (Pelargonium graveolens), 3 drops Clary Sage Oil (Salvia sclarea), 30ml Argan Oil (Argania spinosa)

Process: Combine Geranium and Clary Sage oils with Argan Oil in a bottle. Ideal for balancing emotions and easing tension during massage therapy.

Synergistic Blends for Emotional Support

Comforting Heart Blend

P.T.: 5 minutes

Ingr.: 4 drops Bergamot Oil (Citrus bergamia), 3 drops Rose Oil (Rosa damascena), 2 drops Sandalwood Oil (Santalum album), 30ml Fractionated Coconut Oil (Cocos nucifera)

Process: Mix Bergamot, Rose, and Sandalwood oils with Fractionated Coconut Oil in a small bottle. Apply to the chest area and wrists during times of emotional stress or heartache for comfort.

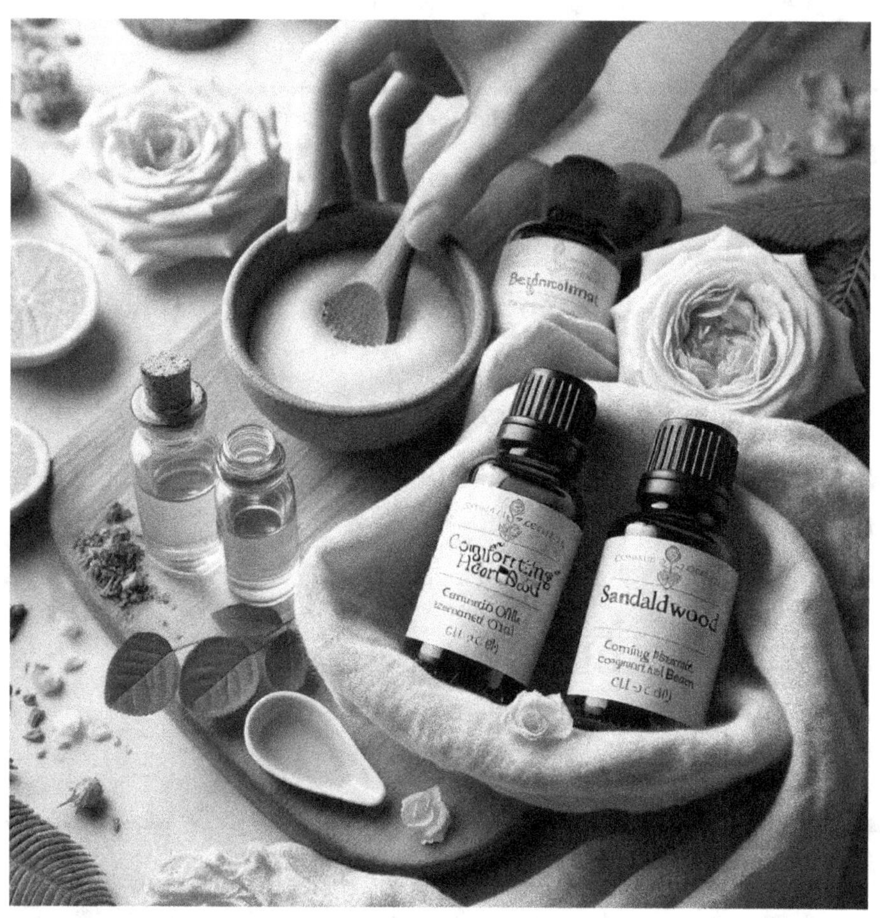

Mind Clarity Mix

P.T.: 4 minutes

Ingr.: 3 drops Peppermint Oil (Mentha piperita), 3 drops Lemon Oil (Citrus limon), 2 drops Rosemary Oil (Rosmarinus officinalis), 30ml Grapeseed Oil (Vitis vinifera)

Process: Blend Peppermint, Lemon, and Rosemary oils with Grapeseed Oil. Use for a temple and neck massage to enhance focus and clear mental fog.

Soothing Sleep Elixir

P.T.: 5 minutes

Ingr.: 5 drops Lavender Oil (Lavandula angustifolia), 2 drops Chamomile Oil (Matricaria chamomilla), 1 drop Vetiver Oil (Vetiveria zizanioides), 30ml Almond Oil (Prunus dulcis)

Process: Combine Lavender, Chamomile, and Vetiver oils with Almond Oil. Massage onto the soles of the feet or diffuse at bedtime for a restful sleep.

Uplift and Balance Aroma

P.T.: 4 minutes

Ingr.: 3 drops Ylang Ylang Oil (Cananga odorata), 3 drops Orange Oil (Citrus sinensis), 2 drops Frankincense Oil (Boswellia carterii), 30ml Jojoba Oil (Simmondsia chinensis)

Process: Mix Ylang Ylang, Orange, and Frankincense oils with Jojoba Oil. Apply to pulse points or use in a diffuser to uplift mood and bring emotional balance.

Stress Relief Synergy

P.T.: 5 minutes

Ingr.: 4 drops Geranium Oil (Pelargonium graveolens), 3 drops Clary Sage Oil (Salvia sclarea), 2 drops Patchouli Oil (Pogostemon cablin), 30ml Argan Oil (Argania spinosa)
Process: Blend Geranium, Clary Sage, and Patchouli oils with Argan Oil. Apply to the back of the neck and shoulders to relieve stress and tension.

As we conclude our exploration of therapeutic blends, we are left with a deeper appreciation for the healing potential of essential oils. This chapter has provided a comprehensive guide to creating natural remedies and supportive blends, illustrating the powerful impact these oils can have on our physical and emotional health. We have seen how, with thoughtful combination and application, essential oils can be transformed into potent solutions for a range of common ailments and emotional states. The knowledge gained here empowers us to embrace a more natural approach to health and well-being, utilizing the gifts of nature to nurture and heal. The journey through this chapter is a reminder of the harmonious relationship between nature and our own health, encouraging us to integrate these therapeutic blends into our daily lives for enhanced well-being and balance.

Book 4: Advanced Aromatherapy: In-Depth Exploration of Essential Oils

CHAPTER 1: Chemical Constituents and Synergy

Embarking on a journey into the heart of essential oils, we explore the intricate world of their chemical constituents. Here, the focus is on the dynamic interplay of terpenes, phenols, ethers, and esters, each bringing unique therapeutic properties to these aromatic elixirs. Our exploration is not merely scientific; it's an insight into the harmonious synergy that occurs within these compounds, bestowing essential oils with their healing prowess. This understanding goes beyond the molecular, highlighting the art and science that underpin the efficacy of essential oils.

Terpenes and Their Therapeutic Effects

In the intricate world of essential oils, terpenes stand as pivotal compounds, orchestrating a symphony of therapeutic effects. These organic compounds, abundant in the natural world, play a crucial role in the medicinal and aromatic properties of essential oils.

Terpenes are the primary constituents of essential oils, contributing not only to their distinct aromas but also to their diverse therapeutic properties. They are classified based on the number of isoprene units they contain, ranging from monoterpenes, sesquiterpenes, to diterpenes, each category having its unique characteristics and health benefits.

Monoterpenes, the most abundant type of terpenes found in essential oils, are renowned for their uplifting and invigorating effects. Limonene, a classic example found in citrus oils, exudes a refreshing and purifying aroma. Its presence is known to enhance mood, provide immune support, and offer antiviral properties. Another significant monoterpene, pinene, prevalent in pine and fir oils, is celebrated for its ability to promote respiratory health and clarity of mind.

Sesquiterpenes, with their more complex molecular structure, impart deeper, grounding aromas. They are particularly effective in balancing emotions and promoting mental clarity. β-Caryophyllene, found in oils like Clove and Black Pepper, is a sesquiterpene that has garnered attention for its anti-inflammatory and analgesic properties, making it beneficial in managing pain and inflammation.

Diterpenes, though less common in essential oils, possess significant therapeutic attributes. They are known for their stabilizing effects on the body and mind, often contributing to the oils' longevity and efficacy. One such diterpene, cembrene, found in certain conifer oils, has shown potential in supporting cardiovascular health and offering antimicrobial benefits.

The therapeutic effects of terpenes extend far beyond their individual properties, demonstrating a remarkable synergy when blended. This synergy, the harmonious interaction between different compounds, amplifies the overall therapeutic potential of essential oils. For instance, the combination of limonene and pinene can enhance the overall respiratory benefits, providing a more effective remedy for respiratory ailments than either terpene alone.

Understanding the therapeutic effects of terpenes also involves recognizing their influence on the body's physiological systems. For example, monoterpenes are known to interact with the limbic system, the part of the brain involved in emotional and behavioral responses. This interaction explains the mood-enhancing and calming effects of essential oils rich in monoterpenes.

In the realm of alternative and complementary medicine, terpenes are increasingly being acknowledged for their potential in supporting holistic health. Their anti-inflammatory, antimicrobial, and antioxidant properties have made them subjects of interest in scientific research, exploring their role in disease prevention and health promotion.

As we embrace the power of terpenes, it becomes evident that these small yet mighty compounds are key players in the efficacy of essential oils. Their diverse therapeutic effects not only enrich our understanding of plant medicine but also empower us to utilize essential oils more effectively. Through the study and application of terpenes, we tap into a deeper level of natural healing, appreciating the intricate ways in which nature supports our journey toward health and well-being.

Phenols and Their Antiseptic Properties

Phenols, a class of chemical compounds found in essential oils, embody a remarkable confluence of antiseptic properties and therapeutic potential. These compounds, characterized by a hydroxyl group attached to an aromatic benzene ring, are renowned for their potent antimicrobial and antioxidant effects.

The antiseptic properties of phenols make them powerful allies in combating bacteria, viruses, and fungi. One of the most well-known phenols, thymol, found in Thyme essential oil, is acclaimed for its robust antibacterial and antifungal activities. It's this compound that grants Thyme oil its reputation as a formidable disinfectant, widely used in both household cleaning and personal hygiene products. Its ability to eliminate a broad spectrum of pathogens makes it invaluable in natural formulations aimed at sanitizing surfaces and purifying the air.

Another phenolic compound, carvacrol, present in Oregano essential oil, shares similar properties with thymol. Its potent antimicrobial action is particularly effective against strains of bacteria that have developed resistance to conventional antibiotics. This attribute positions carvacrol as a crucial component in the fight against evolving microbial threats, emphasizing the relevance of phenols in contemporary health challenges.

Eugenol, the primary phenol in Clove essential oil, is celebrated for its antiseptic and analgesic properties. Its efficacy in dental care is well-documented, providing relief from toothaches and serving as an active ingredient in various dental products. Eugenol's ability to alleviate pain, coupled with its antimicrobial properties, showcases the dual functionality that phenols often exhibit.

Beyond their antimicrobial attributes, phenols are potent antioxidants, scavenging harmful free radicals in the body. This antioxidant capacity contributes to the protective effects of phenolic-rich essential oils against oxidative stress-related diseases, further extending their therapeutic scope.

The synergy between phenols and other chemical constituents in essential oils enhances their efficacy. For instance, the combination of eugenol and caryophyllene in Clove oil results in a synergistic effect, amplifying its analgesic and anti-inflammatory properties. This synergy is not just a sum of parts; it represents a complex interaction that often yields a more potent therapeutic effect than any single constituent could achieve alone.

The application of phenolic compounds in health and wellness is diverse. In aromatherapy, phenol-rich oils are used for their warming and stimulating properties, beneficial in massage blends for sore muscles and arthritic conditions. In skincare, these oils are valued for their purifying and rejuvenating effects, though their potency necessitates careful dilution to avoid skin irritation.

Understanding the properties of phenols is crucial for their safe and effective use. Due to their potency, essential oils high in phenols should be used with caution, particularly with sensitive populations such as children, the elderly, and those with certain health conditions.

In summary, phenols in essential oils represent a powerful arsenal in natural health care, offering antiseptic, antioxidant, and therapeutic benefits. Their broad-spectrum activity against pathogens, coupled with their synergy with other compounds, makes them invaluable in a world increasingly seeking natural health solutions. As we continue to harness the benefits of these potent molecules, we deepen our connection with nature's pharmacy, appreciating the intricate ways in which it supports our journey towards health and vitality.

Ethers and Esters: The Soothing Molecules

In the aromatic world of essential oils, ethers and esters constitute a class of compounds known for their soothing and harmonizing properties. These chemical constituents, though less discussed than their terpene and phenol counterparts, play a pivotal role in the therapeutic effects of many essential oils. Delving into the nature of ethers and esters reveals a fascinating aspect of plant chemistry that is integral to the holistic properties of essential oils.

Esters, formed through the reaction of an acid with an alcohol, are renowned for their calming and balancing effects. They are commonly found in floral oils such as Lavender (Lavandula angustifolia) and Roman Chamomile (Anthemis nobilis). One of the most well-known esters, linalyl acetate, found abundantly in Lavender oil, is celebrated for its ability to reduce anxiety and promote relaxation. This ester contributes significantly to Lavender's efficacy in soothing the mind, easing tension, and aiding sleep.

Another important ester, geranyl acetate, present in Geranium (Pelargonium graveolens) and Ylang Ylang (Cananga odorata) oils, is valued for its uplifting and balancing action. It plays a key role in harmonizing emotions, making it an excellent choice for mood regulation. Esters are also known for their gentle nature, making them suitable for use with all age groups, including children.

Ethers, characterized by an oxygen atom connected to two alkyl or aryl groups, are less common but equally important. They are known for their antispasmodic and expectorant properties. An example of an ether in essential oils is 1,8-cineole, found in Eucalyptus (Eucalyptus globulus) and

Rosemary (Rosmarinus officinalis). This compound is highly effective in clearing respiratory congestion, making it a go-to component in blends designed for relieving cold and cough symptoms.

The synergy between ethers and esters in certain essential oils enhances their therapeutic properties. For instance, the combination of linalyl acetate (ester) and 1,8-cineole (ether) in Rosemary oil results in a blend that is both calming and helpful for respiratory issues. This synergy is crucial, as it allows for a multifaceted approach to wellness, addressing both physical and emotional health.

Esters and ethers also contribute to the aromatic profile of essential oils. Their scents are often described as soft, fruity, and floral, contributing to the overall sensory experience of aromatherapy. This aspect is important, as the olfactory experience plays a significant role in the emotional and psychological effects of essential oils.

In the context of holistic therapy, esters and ethers are often utilized for their soothing effects on the skin. They are found in skincare formulations for their ability to calm irritation, reduce inflammation, and promote skin healing. This skin-friendly nature makes them a preferred choice in products for sensitive or damaged skin.

Understanding the properties and interactions of ethers and esters is crucial for their effective and safe use in aromatherapy. While they are generally considered safe and gentle, it's essential to understand the specific characteristics of each compound and follow proper dilution guidelines.

In conclusion, ethers and esters are vital constituents that contribute significantly to the therapeutic and aromatic qualities of essential oils. Their soothing, balancing, and healing properties make them indispensable in the practice of aromatherapy. As we continue to explore and understand these molecules, we gain a deeper appreciation for the complexity and synergy of essential oils, reinforcing their role as a powerful tool in natural health and wellness.

CHAPTER 2: Aromatic Science and Research

Venturing into the dynamic and evolving realm of aromatic science, this chapter unfolds a comprehensive exploration of the latest discoveries and critical evaluations in the field of aromatherapy. We embark on a journey that marries the rigor of scientific inquiry with the ancient art of essential oil therapy, offering a deep dive into current research, myth debunking, and foresight into future applications. This narrative weaves together the substantiated benefits and addresses misconceptions, shedding light on how contemporary research both validates and expands upon traditional knowledge. The focus is on bridging the gap between empirical evidence and age-old practices, highlighting the fascinating ways in which essential oils continue to contribute to personal wellness and broader healthcare perspectives.

The Latest in Aromatherapy Research

The realm of aromatic science has recently witnessed significant advancements, particularly in the field of aromatherapy research. This surge in scientific interest has transformed traditional practices into a subject of rigorous academic scrutiny, uncovering the substantial potential of essential oils in modern medicine and holistic health.

A key area of recent research focuses on stress reduction and mental health. Studies involving essential oils such as Lavender (Lavandula angustifolia) and Bergamot (Citrus bergamia) have demonstrated their ability to lower cortisol levels, the body's primary stress hormone. This biochemical shift not only aids in alleviating stress and anxiety but also contributes to overall well-being. The application of these oils has shown notable effectiveness in various settings, from soothing anxiety in dental patients to enhancing sleep quality in individuals with insomnia.

Another vital research domain is the role of essential oils as complementary therapies in pain management. Peppermint (Mentha piperita) oil, for instance, is recognized for its analgesic properties, particularly in the context of headaches and migraines. Its cooling sensation, along with anti-inflammatory effects, presents a natural alternative to conventional pain relief methods. Similarly, the warming properties of Ginger (Zingiber officinale) oil have been explored for their efficacy in addressing symptoms associated with arthritis and muscle pain.

The antimicrobial properties of essential oils have also garnered significant attention. In an era increasingly concerned about antibiotic-resistant bacteria, oils such as Tea

Tree (Melaleuca alternifolia) and Eucalyptus (Eucalyptus globulus) are being researched for their potential to combat various microbial infections. These studies validate traditional uses and open new possibilities, including applications in wound care and as natural preservatives in foods and cosmetics.

Research in the field of oncology has also brought to light the chemopreventive properties of essential oils. Preliminary studies indicate that compounds like limonene, found in citrus oils, may possess cancer-preventing properties. While this area of research is still emerging, it hints at the potential role of essential oils in cancer treatment and prevention strategies.

Additionally, the neuroprotective effects of essential oils are becoming increasingly recognized. Some oils are suggested to have protective effects against neurodegenerative diseases such as Alzheimer's and Parkinson's. For example, Rosemary (Rosmarinus officinalis) oil and its component, 1,8-cineole, are being studied for their potential in enhancing cognitive functions and protecting neural health.

Summarizing, the current wave of research in aromatherapy underscores the extensive and versatile healing attributes of essential oils. These investigations validate long-held anecdotal evidence and pave the way for new scientific discoveries and applications. As research continues to delve into the therapeutic potential of these potent plant extracts, we stand on the brink of a new era in aromatic science. This convergence of tradition and innovation, grounded in nature's wisdom, is shaping a future where essential oils play a pivotal role in advancing human health and wellness.

Debunking Myths: Evidence-Based Practice

In the ever-evolving landscape of aromatherapy, the need for evidence-based practice has never been more critical. The world of essential oils is often clouded by myths and misinformation, making it imperative to distinguish between folklore and scientific fact. This pursuit of truth is not a mere academic exercise but a necessary endeavor to ensure safe and effective use of essential oils.

The first myth that often circulates is the idea that all essential oils are completely safe because they are natural. While it's true that essential oils are derived from plants, their concentrated nature means they can be potent and, in some cases, potentially harmful if misused. For instance, certain oils like Wintergreen (Gaultheria procumbens) and Bitter Almond (Prunus dulcis var. amara) can be toxic if ingested. Research underscores the importance of understanding the chemical composition of each oil and adhering to recommended usage guidelines to prevent adverse reactions.

Another common misconception is that essential oils can replace conventional medicine. While essential oils have remarkable therapeutic benefits and can complement traditional treatments, they are not a panacea. Scientific studies have shown that while some oils may have anti-inflammatory or antimicrobial properties, they should not be used as a substitute for professional medical advice or treatment. The integration of essential oils into healthcare should be viewed as a complementary approach, not a replacement for established medical practices.

The belief that essential oils do not cause allergic reactions is another myth that needs addressing. Like any substance, essential oils can trigger allergic responses in some individuals. For example, oils high in phenols, such as Cinnamon (Cinnamomum zeylanicum) or Clove (Syzygium aromaticum), can cause skin irritation or sensitization over time. Evidence-based research encourages conducting patch tests and diluting oils appropriately to minimize the risk of allergic reactions.

There's also the myth of 'therapeutic grade' as a universally recognized standard for essential oils. This term is often used in marketing, but in reality, there is no regulatory body that defines or enforces such a standard. This highlights the importance of sourcing oils from reputable suppliers who provide detailed information about the oil's origin, extraction method, and chemical composition. Relying on evidence-based resources helps consumers and practitioners make informed decisions about the quality and purity of essential oils.

Finally, the idea that more is always better is a misconception that needs to be addressed. With essential oils, a little goes a long way, and excessive use can lead to adverse effects. Research advocates for moderation and educated use, emphasizing that optimal benefits are often achieved with minimal amounts. For instance, a few drops of Lavender oil are sufficient to induce relaxation, and overuse does not necessarily enhance its efficacy.

Navigating the world of aromatherapy requires a balance of traditional knowledge and modern scientific understanding. By debunking myths and embracing an evidence-based approach, we can harness the full potential of essential oils in a safe and effective manner. This commitment to truth not only enhances the practice of aromatherapy but also ensures that its benefits are realized in a responsible and sustainable way. As we continue to learn and grow in our understanding of these potent natural extracts, we contribute to a more informed and discerning community of essential oil users.

Future Trends in Essential Oil Use

As we venture further into the 21st century, the use of essential oils is poised at a fascinating juncture, blending ancient wisdom with innovative technology. The future of essential oils is being shaped by emerging trends that are grounded in scientific research and driven by a growing demand for natural and holistic health solutions. These trends not only forecast an expansion in the usage of essential oils but also predict a significant evolution in their application and integration into daily life.

One of the most prominent trends is the increased focus on sustainability and ethical sourcing. As consumers become more environmentally conscious, there is a growing demand for essential oils that are produced through sustainable practices. This involves not only the responsible sourcing of raw materials but also ensuring fair trade practices and the preservation of biodiversity. The future will likely see a surge in certification programs and eco-labels that guarantee the sustainable and ethical production of essential oils.

Another trend is the integration of technology in aromatherapy. Technological advancements are revolutionizing the way essential oils are used and experienced. From smart diffusers that can be controlled via smartphones to wearable aromatherapy devices, technology is making the use of essential oils more convenient and customizable. Additionally, advancements in extraction methods and quality testing are enhancing the purity and potency of essential oils, making them more effective than ever.

Personalization and customization are also emerging as key trends. As we gain a deeper understanding of the biochemical makeup of essential oils and their interactions with human physiology, there is a growing interest in creating personalized aromatherapy experiences. This could involve tailoring blends to an individual's specific health needs or even genetic makeup, maximizing the therapeutic benefits of essential oils.

The future also holds potential for the increased use of essential oils in conventional healthcare settings. As more research validates the efficacy of essential oils in clinical scenarios, their integration into practices such as pain management, mental health care, and infection control is anticipated. This trend is not about replacing conventional medicine but about complementing it, offering a more holistic approach to health and wellness.

Research into lesser-known essential oils is another trend that is gaining momentum. While popular oils like Lavender and Tea Tree have been extensively studied, there is a vast array of lesser-known oils with untapped therapeutic potential. Future research is likely to explore these underutilized oils, expanding the aromatic palette and offering new solutions for health and wellness challenges.

In addition to health and wellness, the use of essential oils in consumer products is expected to grow. From natural cosmetics and personal care products to eco-friendly cleaning products, essential oils are being increasingly valued for their natural properties and pleasant aromas. This trend reflects a broader shift towards natural and non-toxic products in response to consumer health concerns.

As we look to the future, the potential of essential oils seems boundless. The convergence of tradition, science, and innovation is paving the way for exciting developments in the field of aromatherapy. These future trends not only promise enhanced effectiveness and accessibility of essential oils but also underscore a deeper commitment to sustainability, personalization, and holistic well-being. As we embrace these trends, we continue the journey of rediscovering nature's essence, weaving it into the fabric of modern life in ways that nurture both the individual and the planet.

CHAPTER 3: Clinical Aromatherapy

Embarking on a journey into the heart of clinical aromatherapy, this exploration delves deep into the transformative power of essential oils within a clinical setting. We navigate through real-life case studies, witnessing the harmonious integration of aromatherapy with traditional medicine, and the meticulous crafting of professional aromatherapy protocols.

Case Studies: Successes and Lessons

The journey of clinical aromatherapy is paved with both remarkable successes and invaluable lessons. As we delve into case studies from various clinical settings, we uncover the profound impact that essential oils can have on health and well-being, along with the crucial insights these experiences offer for future practice.

In a notable case study, a patient with chronic insomnia, resistant to conventional treatment, found relief through a tailored aromatherapy regimen. Lavender oil, renowned for its sedative properties, was diffused in the patient's room at night, resulting in improved sleep quality and duration. This case not only underscores the effectiveness of aromatherapy in managing sleep disorders but also highlights the importance of a patient-centered approach, considering individual preferences and responses to different scents.

Another enlightening case involves the use of essential oils in managing pain and anxiety in cancer patients undergoing chemotherapy. A blend of Frankincense (Boswellia carterii), Myrrh (Commiphora myrrha), and Lemon (Citrus limon) oils, applied topically and used in aromatherapy massages, showed significant reduction in pain and anxiety levels. This example demonstrates the potential of essential oils as adjunct therapies in oncology, providing a complementary approach to alleviate some of the side effects associated with cancer treatments.

A particularly inspiring case study comes from a palliative care setting, where a patient with terminal illness experienced enhanced quality of life through aromatherapy. A blend of Rose (Rosa damascena), Sandalwood (Santalum album), and Bergamot (Citrus bergamia) oils was used to address symptoms such as anxiety, restlessness, and pain. The aromatherapy treatment not only offered physical relief but also brought emotional and spiritual comfort to the patient and their family during a challenging time.

In the context of mental health, a study involving patients with depression highlighted the mood-lifting properties of essential oils. A protocol involving the use of uplifting oils such as Sweet Orange (Citrus sinensis) and Peppermint (Mentha piperita) in combination with counseling and medication saw an improvement in patients' overall mood and outlook. This case study illustrates the potential of aromatherapy as part of a holistic treatment plan for mental health conditions.

However, clinical aromatherapy is not without its challenges and lessons. A case involving an adverse reaction to a potent oil blend serves as a reminder of the importance of safety and proper dilution in aromatherapy practice. It emphasizes the need for thorough knowledge of each oil's properties and potential interactions, especially when dealing with vulnerable populations or individuals with specific health conditions.

These case studies collectively paint a picture of aromatherapy's versatility and effectiveness in clinical settings. They highlight the necessity of integrating traditional medical practices with complementary approaches like aromatherapy, ensuring a well-rounded, patient-centric model of care. Through these stories of healing and learning, we gain not only evidence of the efficacy of essential oils but also insights into their responsible and effective application. As we continue to explore the potential of clinical aromatherapy, these case studies serve as guiding beacons, illuminating the path to a more integrative and compassionate approach to healthcare.

Integrative Approaches with Traditional Medicine

The integration of aromatherapy into traditional medicine marks a significant evolution in healthcare, one that embraces the convergence of ancient wisdom and modern science. This integrative approach, where clinical aromatherapy complements conventional medical practices, is opening new pathways for enhancing patient care and treatment outcomes.

At the forefront of this integration is the recognition of aromatherapy's role in pain management. Traditional pain relief methods, while effective, often come with side effects that can be mitigated by incorporating essential oils. For instance, in post-surgical care, the use of Lavender oil for its analgesic properties has been found to reduce the need for opioid pain relievers, thus minimizing their side effects. This harmonious blend of pharmacology and aromatherapy offers a more holistic approach to pain relief, prioritizing patient comfort and well-being.

In the realm of mental health, the incorporation of essential oils into psychiatric treatment plans is gaining traction. Oils such as Bergamot and Frankincense are being used adjunctively with psychotherapy and pharmacotherapy to alleviate symptoms of depression and anxiety. These oils work not only on a physiological level but also provide psychological comfort, enhancing the overall therapeutic experience.

The potential of essential oils in enhancing the efficacy of antibiotics presents another exciting avenue for integration. Research has shown that certain oils, like Tea Tree and Eucalyptus, possess antimicrobial properties that can complement antibiotic treatments, especially in the case of antibiotic-resistant infections. This synergy between traditional medicine and aromatherapy could play a pivotal role in addressing one of the most pressing challenges in modern healthcare.

Aromatherapy is also finding its place in palliative care, where the quality of life for patients with terminal illnesses is paramount. Here, essential oils are used not only for symptom management but also for providing psychological and spiritual comfort. In hospice settings, aromatherapy protocols are personalized to address individual patient needs, ranging from pain and nausea relief to providing a sense of peace and calm during the end-of-life journey.

In pediatric care, the gentle nature of certain essential oils, such as Roman Chamomile and Mandarin, is being utilized to soothe common ailments in children, such as colic and sleep disturbances. This integration acknowledges the need for gentler, non-invasive treatment options in pediatric medicine, offering effective remedies that are both safe and comforting for younger patients.

Furthermore, the collaboration between aromatherapists and healthcare professionals is fostering a more comprehensive approach to patient care. Through this collaboration, tailored aromatherapy protocols are being developed, taking into account the patient's medical history, current treatments, and specific health needs. This bespoke approach ensures that aromatherapy is not only complementary but also coherent with the patient's overall treatment plan.

The integration of clinical aromatherapy with traditional medicine is not without its challenges. It requires an ongoing effort to educate healthcare professionals about the benefits and safe application of essential oils. Additionally, it calls for rigorous research to further validate the efficacy of aromatherapy in clinical settings.

In essence, the integrative approach in clinical aromatherapy represents a significant stride towards a more holistic and patient-centric model of healthcare. It acknowledges the multifaceted nature of health and wellness, respecting both the scientific rigor of traditional medicine and the holistic benefits of aromatherapy. As this integration continues to evolve, it holds the promise of transforming healthcare practices, offering patients a harmonious blend of the best of both worlds.

Creating Professional Aromatherapy Protocols

In the realm of clinical aromatherapy, the creation of professional protocols stands as a cornerstone for ensuring safe, effective, and consistent practices. These protocols are not mere guidelines but structured methodologies that integrate the art of aromatherapy into the science of healing. Crafting such protocols involves a comprehensive understanding of essential oil properties, patient assessment, and the nuances of therapeutic application.

The foundation of any professional aromatherapy protocol begins with a thorough grasp of essential oil chemistry. Each oil's unique chemical makeup determines its therapeutic properties, safety concerns, and methods of application. For instance, understanding that oils high in monoterpenes are generally uplifting and stimulating, while those rich in sesquiterpenes are more grounding, guides the aromatherapist in selecting the right oil for each individual's needs.

Patient assessment is another critical aspect of protocol development. This process involves more than just an understanding of the patient's present ailment; it delves into their medical history, current medications, allergies, and overall health. Such detailed assessment ensures that the chosen essential oils complement the patient's condition without causing adverse interactions. For example, a patient with hypertension would require a different approach than someone with a respiratory condition, guiding the selection and concentration of oils used.

Determining the method of application is a crucial step in protocol development. Essential oils can be administered in various ways - inhalation, topical application, or diffusion, to name a few. Each method has its benefits and considerations. For instance, inhalation is effective for respiratory or emotional issues, while topical applications are more suited for localized pain or skin conditions. The protocol must specify the method that aligns best with the therapeutic objectives and patient preferences.

Dosage and dilution are vital components of any aromatherapy protocol. The potency of essential oils necessitates careful consideration of the concentration used. This is particularly important for vulnerable populations like children, the elderly, or those with sensitive skin. Professional protocols dictate precise dilution ratios to maximize therapeutic benefits while minimizing risks.

The frequency and duration of treatment are also pivotal elements of aromatherapy protocols. These factors depend on the ailment being treated, the patient's response to the therapy, and the specific oils being used. A protocol might recommend a more frequent application for acute conditions and a gradual tapering for chronic issues, always with an eye on the patient's feedback and progress.

Professional protocols also encompass safety guidelines, which are paramount in clinical aromatherapy. These guidelines cover everything from contraindications and potential oil interactions to proper storage and handling of essential oils. They serve as a safeguard against misuse and ensure that aromatherapy is practiced with the utmost care and responsibility.

In addition to these technical aspects, creating professional aromatherapy protocols also involves an understanding of the holistic nature of aromatherapy. It's about recognizing that each patient is a unique individual, requiring a tailored approach that addresses not just their physical symptoms but their emotional and spiritual well-being. This holistic perspective is what sets clinical aromatherapy apart and makes it a deeply personal and transformative healing practice.

In essence, the development of professional aromatherapy protocols is a meticulous and thoughtful process. It requires a blend of scientific knowledge, clinical experience, and a deep respect for the natural power of essential oils. As the field of clinical aromatherapy continues to grow, these protocols will serve as vital tools, guiding practitioners in offering safe, effective, and compassionate care to those seeking relief and healing through the art and science of essential oils.

Concluding our exploration of clinical aromatherapy, we emerge with a richer understanding of the impactful role essential oils play in the realm of healthcare. The journey through case studies, integrative practices, and protocol development paints a comprehensive picture of how aromatherapy can be expertly woven into clinical settings. It emphasizes the importance of evidence-based, personalized approaches in maximizing the therapeutic potential of essential oils. This chapter not only affirms the efficacy and versatility of aromatherapy in clinical applications but also underscores the necessity for continued research and education in this field. As we reflect on these insights, it becomes clear that clinical aromatherapy, with its unique blend of tradition and innovation, is poised to make significant contributions to holistic healthcare, enriching the lives of those seeking natural paths to healing and well-being.

CHAPTER 4: The Business of Essential Oils

Embarking on the Business of Essential Oils, this chapter unveils the complex yet rewarding journey of establishing a successful essential oil venture. It begins by exploring the vital importance of ethical sourcing and sustainability, emphasizing that these are not mere trends but essential practices for the health of our planet and the purity of the products. The narrative then transitions to the artistry of building an aromatherapy brand, highlighting the significance of creating a resonant story and a meaningful connection with consumers. The chapter also delves into the intricate web of navigating regulations and compliance, underscoring its critical role in ensuring business integrity and customer safety. Each section is woven together to provide entrepreneurs with a holistic view of the industry, from the ground up, showcasing how to build a brand that is not just financially successful but also ethically sound and environmentally conscious.

Ethical Sourcing and Sustainability in the Essential Oil Industry

In the burgeoning field of essential oils, the principles of ethical sourcing and sustainability stand as foundational pillars, integral to the integrity and future of the industry. This commitment extends beyond mere business practices; it is a testament to respect for the earth and its resources, a pledge to uphold the balance between human needs and environmental stewardship.

Ethical sourcing in the essential oil industry is a multifaceted endeavor, involving conscientious decisions at every step, from plant cultivation to oil extraction. It begins with the selection of source plants. Sustainable practices dictate that these plants should be grown in environments where they thrive naturally, minimizing ecological disruption. By choosing indigenous species and implementing organic farming methods, producers can contribute to biodiversity conservation and prevent soil degradation and water contamination. This approach also ensures the highest quality of essential oils, as plants grown in their native habitats possess optimal chemical profiles.

The harvesting process further underscores the importance of ethical sourcing. It is imperative to harvest plants in a manner that does not deplete natural populations or harm the local ecosystem. Sustainable harvesting involves picking only what is needed, leaving enough plant material for regeneration. In some cases, it means waiting for the right stage of plant growth to ensure sustainability. Such practices not only preserve plant species for future generations but also maintain the ecological balance within the harvesting area.

The extraction of essential oils is another critical area where sustainability plays a key role. Traditional extraction methods, like steam distillation, should be carried out with energy efficiency and water conservation in mind. The use of renewable energy sources, such as solar or wind power, and the recycling of water in the distillation process are steps toward more sustainable practices. Additionally, responsible companies are exploring innovative extraction methods that are both environmentally friendly and capable of yielding high-quality oils.

The ethical aspect of sourcing also encompasses fair trade practices. It is about ensuring that the farmers and harvesters who are the backbone of the essential oil industry receive fair compensation for their labor. Fair trade practices help uplift local communities, providing them with a sustainable livelihood and improving their quality of life. By investing in these communities, companies can help preserve traditional knowledge and practices that are invaluable to the industry.

Sustainability in the essential oil industry is not a static goal but a continuous journey. It involves constant assessment and adaptation of practices to meet evolving environmental challenges. This journey requires collaboration between farmers, producers, scientists, and consumers. By educating consumers about the value of ethically sourced and sustainable products, companies can create a market that supports these practices. Consumers, in turn, become active participants in this endeavor, their choices shaping the future of the industry.

In essence, ethical sourcing and sustainability in the essential oil industry are more than business strategies; they are moral imperatives. They reflect a deep reverence for nature and a commitment to preserving its bounty for future generations. As the industry grows, this commitment must remain at its heart, guiding decisions and shaping practices. It is a path of respect, responsibility, and vision, leading toward a future where business and nature exist in harmonious synergy.

Building an Aromatherapy Brand

In the realm of aromatherapy, building a brand transcends the mere selling of essential oils and related products. It's about crafting a story, an experience that resonates deeply with the consumers, connecting them not just to a product but to a lifestyle, a philosophy. Creating an aromatherapy brand is an artful journey, one that intertwines the aromatic essences of nature with the essence of the brand's identity.

The cornerstone of building a successful aromatherapy brand lies in understanding the heart and soul of aromatherapy itself. It's more than just understanding the products; it's about embracing the holistic approach to wellness that aromatherapy represents. This requires a deep knowledge of the therapeutic properties of essential oils, their blends, and applications. A brand with a solid foundation in the science and art of aromatherapy can develop products that are not only effective but also steeped in authenticity.

The identity of an aromatherapy brand is often reflected in its storytelling. How a brand narrates its journey, its commitment to quality, and its dedication to wellness can create a lasting impression. Storytelling is a powerful tool that can weave together the brand's philosophy, its ethical sourcing practices, its commitment to sustainability, and the quality of its products into a cohesive narrative. This narrative should speak to the heart, evoking emotions and building a connection that goes beyond the transactional.

A key aspect of building an aromatherapy brand is the aesthetic presentation. This encompasses everything from product design, packaging, and labeling to the overall visual theme of the brand. The aesthetic should mirror the brand's ethos. For instance, a brand focusing on purity and natural ingredients might opt for clean, minimalistic packaging, using materials that are eco-friendly and sustainable. The visual appeal is often the first point of contact with the consumer, and it sets the tone for their experience with the brand.

Engaging with the community is another vital element. In today's digital age, creating an online presence where the brand can interact with its audience, share valuable content, and build a community is essential. Social media platforms, blogs, and forums provide opportunities not just for marketing but for education and engagement. Through these channels, a brand can share the knowledge of aromatherapy, tips for wellness, and stories behind the products, fostering a community of informed and loyal customers.

Innovation is the fuel that drives a brand forward. The aromatherapy market is dynamic, with evolving consumer needs and preferences. Staying ahead of the curve with innovative products, unique blends, or new applications of essential oils can distinguish a brand in a crowded marketplace. However, innovation should always be aligned with the brand's core values and mission.

Finally, customer experience is paramount. From the first interaction to the post-purchase phase, every touchpoint is an opportunity to leave a positive impression. Exceptional customer service, transparent communication, and a willingness to listen and respond to customer feedback can elevate a brand significantly.

In essence, building an aromatherapy brand is about crafting a holistic experience. It's about establishing a connection that transcends the physical products and taps into the emotional and spiritual well-being of the consumers. It's a journey that requires passion, knowledge, authenticity, and a relentless pursuit of excellence. In the landscape of aromatherapy, such a brand becomes not just a choice but a companion in the journey of wellness.

Navigating Regulations and Compliance in the Essential Oil Industry

In the essential oil industry, navigating the complex web of regulations and compliance is a crucial aspect that brands must master to ensure not only the legality of their operations but also the safety and trust of their consumers. This process is intricate, involving various levels of legislation and oversight, both locally and globally. Understanding and adhering to these regulations is not just a legal obligation; it's a commitment to quality and integrity.

The first step in navigating these regulatory waters is understanding the diverse landscape of laws that govern the industry. This includes regulations from bodies such as the

Food and Drug Administration (FDA) in the United States, the European Medicines Agency (EMA) in Europe, and other international entities. These organizations set standards for product safety, labeling, and marketing claims. For instance, the FDA regulates essential oils differently based on their intended use - whether as cosmetics, drugs, or dietary supplements. Each classification has its own set of rules regarding production, labeling, and advertising.

Labeling is a critical area of focus. Mislabeling or making unfounded claims can lead to severe penalties. It's imperative for brands to be precise and compliant in their labeling. This means accurately listing ingredients, avoiding claims that could classify the product as a drug (unless approved as such), and providing necessary warnings and usage instructions. Transparency in labeling not only complies with legal standards but also builds consumer trust.

Another aspect is the compliance with Good Manufacturing Practices (GMP). These are guidelines that ensure products are consistently produced and controlled according to quality standards. GMP covers all aspects of production, from the raw materials, facilities, and equipment to the training and personal hygiene of staff. Adherence to GMP is essential not only for compliance but for ensuring the consistency and quality of the essential oils.

Compliance also extends to environmental regulations. With increasing awareness and concern over environmental impact, brands must ensure their sourcing, manufacturing, and distribution practices are environmentally responsible and sustainable. This includes adherence to laws governing the sourcing of raw materials, waste disposal, emissions, and more. These practices are not just about avoiding legal repercussions; they are about committing to the planet's health and future generations.

For international brands, compliance becomes even more complex. They must navigate the laws of each country in which they operate. This requires a deep understanding of international trade laws, tariffs, and customs regulations. It's a delicate balance of maintaining global brand consistency while adapting to local regulations and cultural nuances.

Staying informed and agile is key in this ever-evolving regulatory landscape. Laws and guidelines can change, and it's essential for brands to remain vigilant and adaptable. This may involve working with legal experts, staying updated through industry associations, and actively participating in regulatory discussions and forums.

In conclusion, navigating regulations and compliance in the essential oil industry is a multifaceted and ongoing process. It requires diligence, knowledge, and a commitment to excellence and integrity. By mastering this aspect, brands not only protect themselves legally but also elevate their standing in the eyes of their consumers and the industry at large. It's a testament to their dedication to quality, safety, and ethical responsibility.

Book 5: The Aromatherapist's Kitchen: Crafting Your Own Essential Oil Creations

CHAPTER 1: The Art of Blending

Delving into the aromatic world of essential oils, this chapter opens a window to the art of blending, a skill combining creativity with scientific understanding. It reveals the complexities and joys of creating unique essential oil blends, each with its own character and therapeutic benefit. Readers are guided through the nuances of crafting balanced blends, formulating signature scents, and tailoring aromas for seasonal wellbeing. This journey is about more than just mixing oils; it's an exploration of how these blends can influence emotions, health, and the atmosphere of our surroundings. The art of blending is presented as a harmonious fusion of knowledge and intuition, where each combination of scents can tell a story, evoke a mood, or bring a sense of comfort.

Crafting Balanced Blends

Tranquil Meadow Blend

P.T.: 10 minutes

Ingr.: 5 drops Lavender Oil (Lavandula angustifolia), 3 drops Clary Sage Oil (Salvia sclarea), 2 drops Ylang Ylang Oil (Cananga odorata)

Process: In a small amber bottle, combine Lavender, Clary Sage, and Ylang Ylang oils. Shake gently to blend. Ideal for diffusing in the evening for a calming and soothing atmosphere.

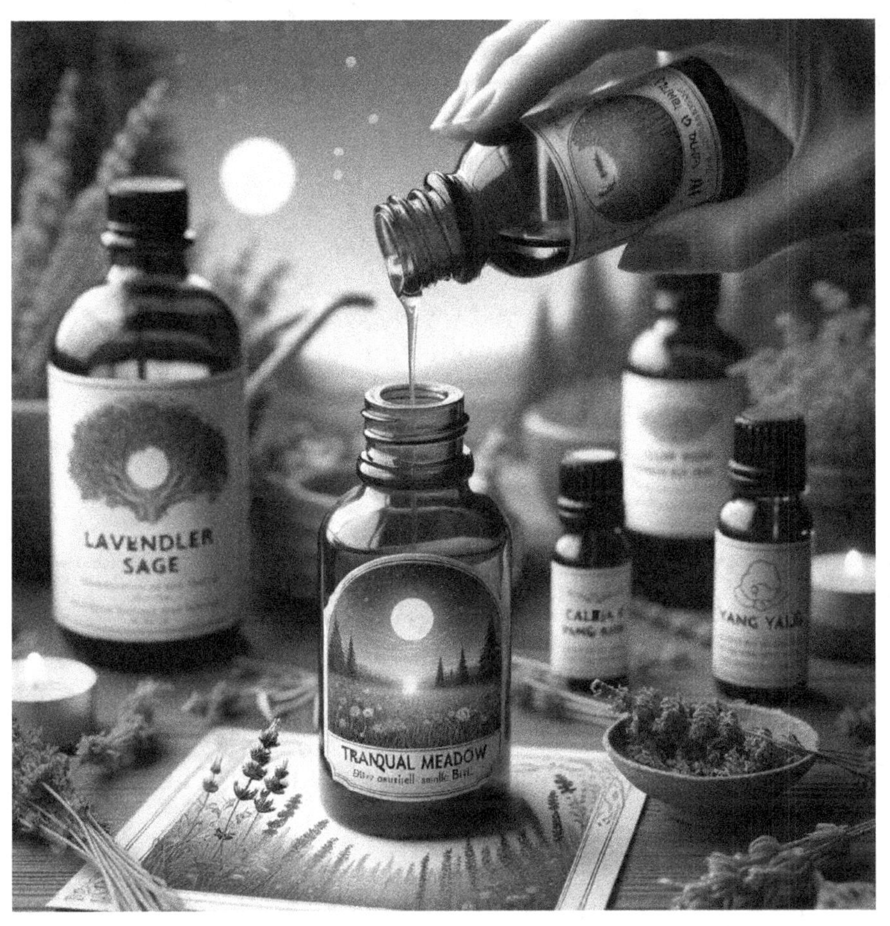

Morning Vitality Elixir

P.T.: 8 minutes

Ingr.: 4 drops Lemon Oil (Citrus limon), 4 drops Peppermint Oil (Mentha piperita), 2 drops Rosemary Oil (Rosmarinus officinalis)

Process: Blend Lemon, Peppermint, and Rosemary oils in a dark glass bottle. Shake well. Use in a morning diffuser to invigorate the senses and kickstart the day.

Forest Retreat Aura

P.T.: 10 minutes

Ingr.: 5 drops Pine Oil (Pinus sylvestris), 3 drops Cedarwood Oil (Cedrus atlantica), 2 drops Juniper Berry Oil (Juniperus communis)

Process: Mix Pine, Cedarwood, and Juniper Berry oils in a bottle. Shake to combine. Diffuse to create a refreshing, forest-like ambiance, ideal for meditation or relaxation.

Harmonious Zen Blend

P.T.: 7 minutes

Ingr.: 4 drops Frankincense Oil (Boswellia carterii), 4 drops Myrrh Oil (Commiphora myrrha), 2 drops Patchouli Oil (Pogostemon cablin)

Process: In a small blending bottle, combine Frankincense, Myrrh, and Patchouli oils. Gently mix. This blend is perfect for grounding and spiritual connection during yoga or quiet reflection.

Citrus Blossom Zest

P.T.: 9 minutes

Ingr.: 5 drops Sweet Orange Oil (Citrus sinensis), 3 drops Grapefruit Oil (Citrus paradisi), 2 drops Neroli Oil (Citrus aurantium)

Process: Add Sweet Orange, Grapefruit, and Neroli oils to a blend bottle. Shake to integrate the oils. Ideal for uplifting the mood and freshening up living spaces during the day.

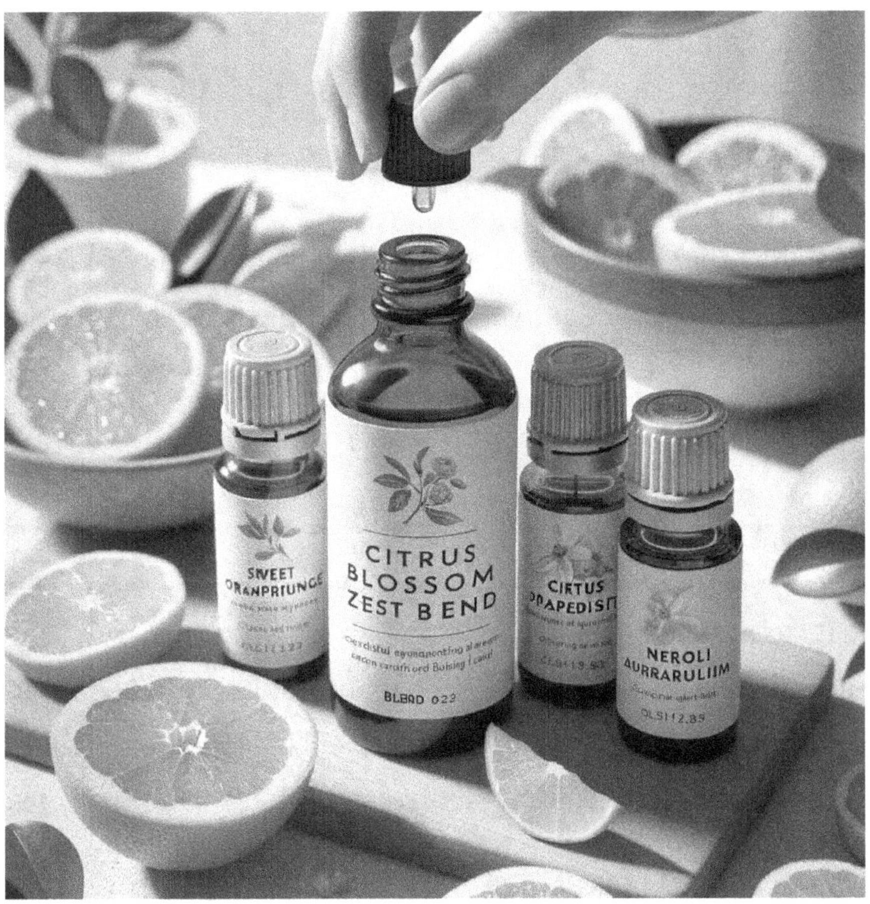

Creating Signature Scents

Elegant Evening Whisper

P.T.: 12 minutes

Ingr.: 4 drops Jasmine Oil (Jasminum officinale), 3 drops Sandalwood Oil (Santalum album), 2 drops Vanilla Oil (Vanilla planifolia)

Process: Combine Jasmine, Sandalwood, and Vanilla oils in an amber glass bottle. Gently swirl to blend the oils. This scent is perfect for evenings, creating an elegant and romantic atmosphere.

Zesty Citrus Grove

P.T.: 10 minutes

Ingr.: 5 drops Bergamot Oil (Citrus bergamia), 3 drops Lime Oil (Citrus aurantifolia), 2 drops Basil Oil (Ocimum basilicum)

Process: In a small bottle, mix Bergamot, Lime, and Basil oils. Shake well to unify the scents. Use in a diffuser for a refreshing and uplifting daytime aroma that invigorates any space.

Mystic Forest Essence

P.T.: 11 minutes

Ingr.: 4 drops Fir Needle Oil (Abies sibirica), 3 drops Cypress Oil (Cupressus sempervirens), 3 drops Black Spruce Oil (Picea mariana)

Process: Blend Fir Needle, Cypress, and Black Spruce oils in a dark bottle. Shake to combine. Ideal for creating a mystic forest ambiance, reminiscent of a serene woodland.

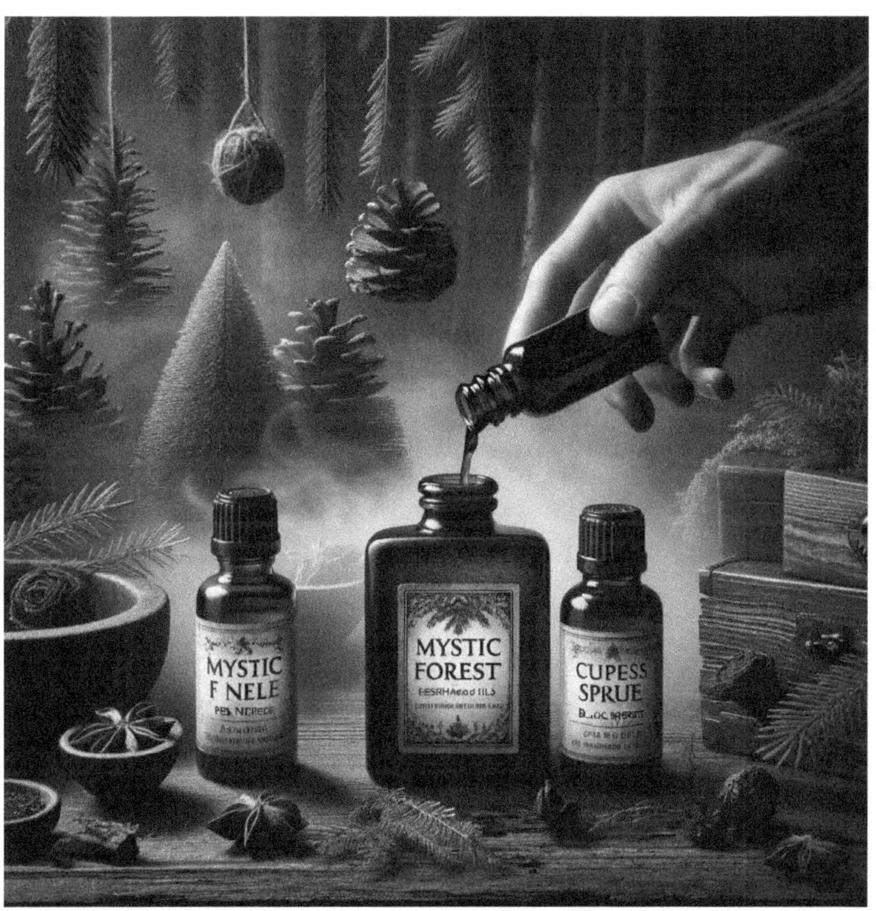

Sunset Serenity Charm

P.T.: 9 minutes

Ingr.: 4 drops Lavender Oil (Lavandula angustifolia), 3 drops Clary Sage Oil (Salvia sclarea), 2 drops Geranium Oil (Pelargonium graveolens)

Process: Mix Lavender, Clary Sage, and Geranium oils in a blending vessel. Carefully shake the bottle. This blend is wonderful for unwinding in the late afternoon or early evening, offering a serene transition to nighttime.

Ocean Breeze Euphoria

P.T.: 8 minutes

Ingr.: 5 drops Sea Fennel Oil (Crithmum maritimum), 3 drops Yuzu Oil (Citrus junos), 2 drops Peppermint Oil (Mentha piperita)

Process: Combine Sea Fennel, Yuzu, and Peppermint oils in a glass container. Gently mix. Ideal for mimicking a refreshing ocean breeze, this scent is great for revitalizing mornings or afternoons.

Seasonal Blends for Home and Health

Autumn Harvest Delight

P.T.: 10 minutes

Ingr.: 5 drops Cinnamon Bark Oil (Cinnamomum verum), 4 drops Sweet Orange Oil (Citrus sinensis), 2 drops Clove Bud Oil (Syzygium aromaticum)

Process: In a small amber bottle, blend Cinnamon Bark, Sweet Orange, and Clove Bud oils. Shake well to mix. This blend is perfect for diffusing in the autumn months, creating a warm, inviting atmosphere reminiscent of fall harvests.

Winter Wonderland Whisper

P.T.: 12 minutes

Ingr.: 4 drops Peppermint Oil (Mentha piperita), 3 drops Fir Needle Oil (Abies sibirica), 3 drops Cedarwood Oil (Cedrus atlantica)

Process: Combine Peppermint, Fir Needle, and Cedarwood oils in a dark glass bottle. Gently swirl to blend. Ideal for the winter season, this scent brings a refreshing and cozy feeling, like a serene winter forest.

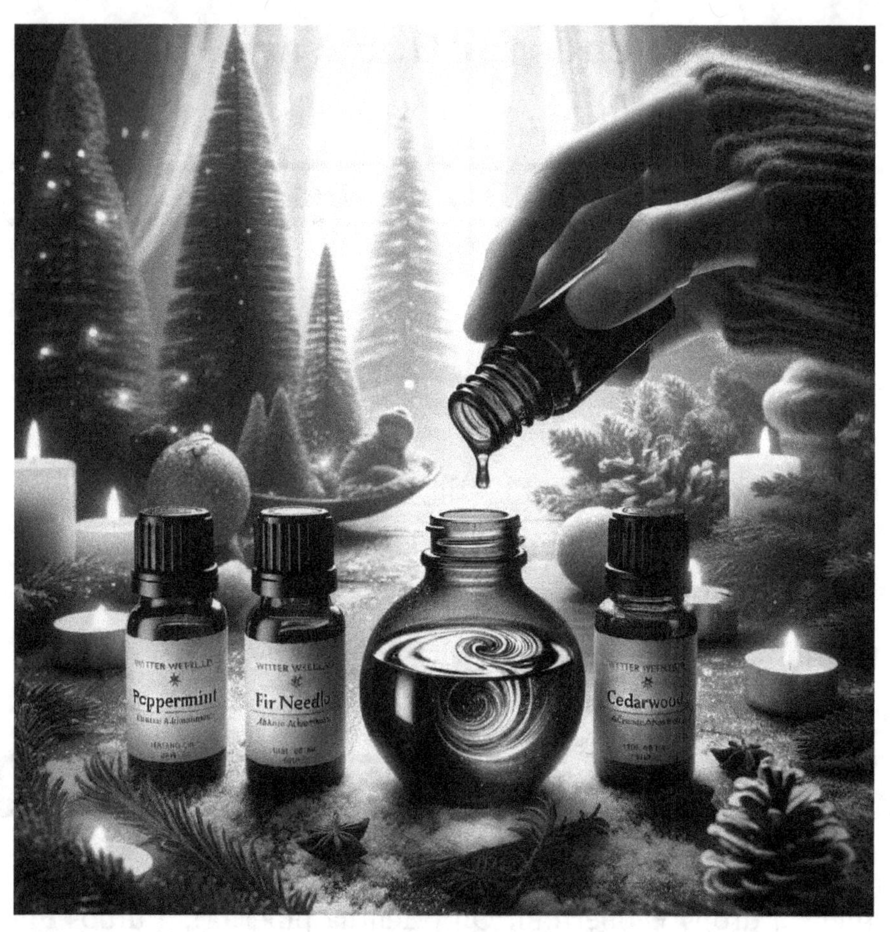

Spring Blossom Breeze

P.T.: 8 minutes

Ingr.: 5 drops Lemon Oil (Citrus limon), 3 drops Geranium Oil (Pelargonium graveolens), 2 drops Jasmine Oil (Jasminum officinale)

Process: Mix Lemon, Geranium, and Jasmine oils in a blending vessel. Shake well. Perfect for welcoming the spring, this blend offers a fresh, floral scent that evokes blooming gardens.

Summer Solstice Aura

P.T.: 9 minutes

Ingr.: 5 drops Bergamot Oil (Citrus bergamia), 3 drops Lavender Oil (Lavandula angustifolia), 2 drops Ylang Ylang Oil (Cananga odorata)

Process: In a small bottle, combine Bergamot, Lavender, and Ylang Ylang oils. Shake to integrate. Suitable for the summer months, this blend has a light, uplifting aroma perfect for long, sunny days.

Rainy Day Reflection

P.T.: 11 minutes

Ingr.: 4 drops Vetiver Oil (Vetiveria zizanioides), 3 drops Lemon Oil (Citrus limon), 3 drops Eucalyptus Oil (Eucalyptus globulus)

Process: Blend Vetiver, Lemon, and Eucalyptus oils in a dark glass container. Shake gently. Ideal for rainy days, this blend provides a comforting, refreshing scent that enhances indoor ambiance.

As we conclude our journey through the art of blending, we emerge with a deeper understanding and appreciation for this intricate craft. This chapter has illuminated the vast possibilities that lie in combining essential oils, from creating harmonious blends for daily use to capturing the essence of seasons in a bottle. The insights gathered here equip us with the knowledge to experiment and craft our own blends, tailored to personal preferences and specific needs. This exploration underlines blending as an enriching practice, where creativity meets the therapeutic wonders of nature. Armed with these techniques, we are inspired to continue experimenting, discovering, and enjoying the endless combinations and benefits that the world of essential oils has to offer.

CHAPTER 2: Specialty Topical Applications

Embarking on a journey through the world of specialty topical applications, this chapter reveals the art of creating natural, therapeutic formulations for the skin. From healing salves and balms that soothe and repair, to luxurious lotions and butters that hydrate and nourish, each section unfolds the secrets of crafting these potent remedies. The chapter further delves into the realm of therapeutic gels and serums, offering insights into their preparation for targeted skincare needs. Emphasizing the use of natural ingredients and essential oils, these recipes are not just skincare products; they are a fusion of nature's best, designed to enhance skin health and overall well-being. This exploration is an invitation to embrace the power of handcrafted, personalized skincare, offering effective, natural alternatives to commercial products.

Healing Salves and Balms

Soothing Lavender-Chamomile Balm

P.T.: 20 minutes

Ingr.: 2 tbsp Beeswax pellets, 4 tbsp Coconut oil, 1 tbsp Shea butter, 10 drops Lavender essential oil, 10 drops Chamomile essential oil

Process: Melt beeswax, coconut oil, and shea butter in a double boiler. Once melted, remove from heat. Cool slightly and stir in Lavender and Chamomile essential oils. Pour into a small jar and let set until solid.

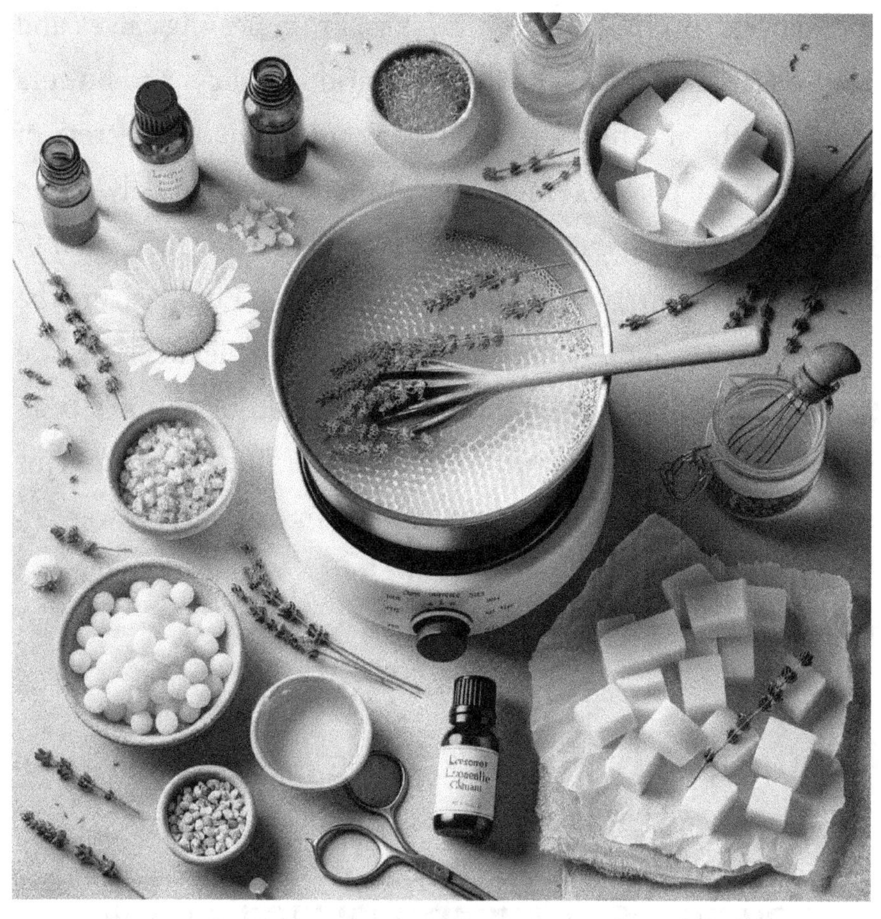

Herbal Rescue Salve

P.T.: 30 minutes

Ingr.: 3 tbsp Calendula-infused Olive oil, 2 tbsp Jojoba oil, 2 tbsp Beeswax, 5 drops Tea Tree oil, 5 drops Eucalyptus oil

Process: Gently heat the Calendula-infused Olive oil, Jojoba oil, and Beeswax in a double boiler until the beeswax melts. Remove from heat, add Tea Tree and Eucalyptus oils, and mix well. Pour into tins and allow to cool and solidify.

Calming Rose Salve

P.T.: 25 minutes

Ingr.: 2 tbsp Almond oil, 1 tbsp Beeswax, 1/2 tbsp Rosehip oil, 10 drops Rose essential oil, 5 drops Geranium oil

Process: Heat Almond oil and beeswax in a double boiler until melted. Remove from heat, add Rosehip oil, Rose and Geranium essential oils. Stir and pour into small jars. Let it set until firm.

Minty Eucalyptus Muscle Balm

P.T.: 20 minutes

Ingr.: 3 tbsp Cocoa butter, 2 tbsp Sweet Almond oil, 2 tbsp Beeswax, 10 drops Eucalyptus oil, 10 drops Peppermint oil

Process: Melt Cocoa butter, Sweet Almond oil, and Beeswax together over a double boiler. Once melted, remove from heat, add Eucalyptus and Peppermint oils, and stir well. Pour into containers and allow to cool.

Citrus Bliss Healing Balm

P.T.: 22 minutes

Ingr.: 2 tbsp Shea butter, 1 tbsp Mango butter, 2 tbsp Beeswax, 5 drops Lemon oil, 5 drops Orange oil, 5 drops Grapefruit oil

Process: Combine Shea butter, Mango butter, and Beeswax in a double boiler and melt them together. Remove from heat, then add Lemon, Orange, and Grapefruit essential oils. Stir well and pour into jars. Allow to set until solid.

Luxurious Lotions and Butters

Velvet Rose Hydration Butter

P.T.: 25 minutes

Ingr.: 1/2 cup Shea butter, 1/4 cup Coconut oil, 2 tbsp Rosehip oil, 15 drops Rose essential oil, 10 drops Geranium oil

Process: Whip Shea butter and Coconut oil in a bowl until creamy. Gradually mix in Rosehip oil. Add Rose and Geranium essential oils, continuing to whip until light and fluffy. Store in a cool, dry place.

Citrus Glow Body Lotion

P.T.: 30 minutes

Ingr.: 1/2 cup Aloe Vera gel, 1/4 cup Sweet Almond oil, 1 tbsp Beeswax, 10 drops Lemon oil, 10 drops Orange oil

Process: Melt Beeswax and Sweet Almond oil over a double boiler. Remove from heat and let cool slightly. Slowly add Aloe Vera gel while whisking. Stir in Lemon and Orange essential oils. Pour into a container and allow to set.

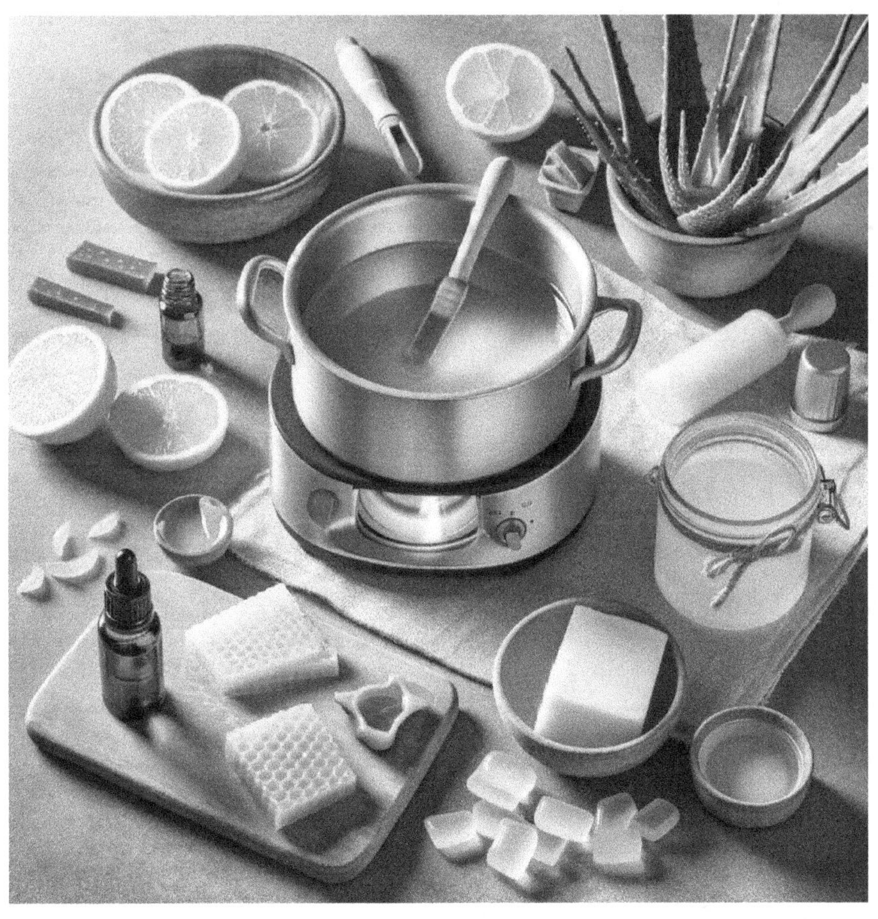

Soothing Lavender Body Butter

P.T.: 20 minutes

Ingr.: 1/2 cup Cocoa butter, 1/4 cup Jojoba oil, 15 drops Lavender oil, 5 drops Chamomile oil

Process: Gently melt Cocoa butter and Jojoba oil in a double boiler. Once melted, remove from heat and cool slightly. Add Lavender and Chamomile essential oils. Whip until the mixture is fluffy. Store in a jar.

Minty Eucalyptus Refreshing Butter

P.T.: 22 minutes

Ingr.: 1/2 cup Mango butter, 1/4 cup Grapeseed oil, 10 drops Peppermint oil, 10 drops Eucalyptus oil

Process: Melt Mango butter and Grapeseed oil in a double boiler. Remove from heat and allow to cool. Stir in Peppermint and Eucalyptus oils. Whip until airy and light. Keep in an airtight container.

Exotic Jasmine and Ylang-Ylang Body Cream

P.T.: 35 minutes

Ingr.: 1/2 cup Kokum butter, 1/4 cup Argan oil, 15 drops Jasmine oil, 10 drops Ylang Ylang oil

Process: Melt Kokum butter in a double boiler, then blend in Argan oil. After removing from heat, cool slightly before adding Jasmine and Ylang Ylang essential oils. Whip until it reaches a creamy consistency. Transfer to a container for storage.

Therapeutic Gels and Serums

Radiant Skin Antioxidant Serum

P.T.: 15 minutes

Ingr.: 1/4 cup Jojoba oil, 1 tbsp Vitamin E oil, 10 drops Frankincense oil, 10 drops Carrot Seed oil

Process: Mix Jojoba oil and Vitamin E oil in a small bowl. Add Frankincense and Carrot Seed essential oils, blending well. Pour the mixture into a dark glass dropper bottle. Apply a few drops to the face and neck after cleansing, morning and night.

Soothing Aloe Vera Gel for Irritated Skin

P.T.: 10 minutes

Ingr.: 1/2 cup Aloe Vera gel, 10 drops Lavender oil, 5 drops Chamomile oil

Process: In a mixing bowl, combine Aloe Vera gel with Lavender and Chamomile essential oils. Transfer to an airtight container. Apply to irritated or sunburnt skin for a soothing effect.

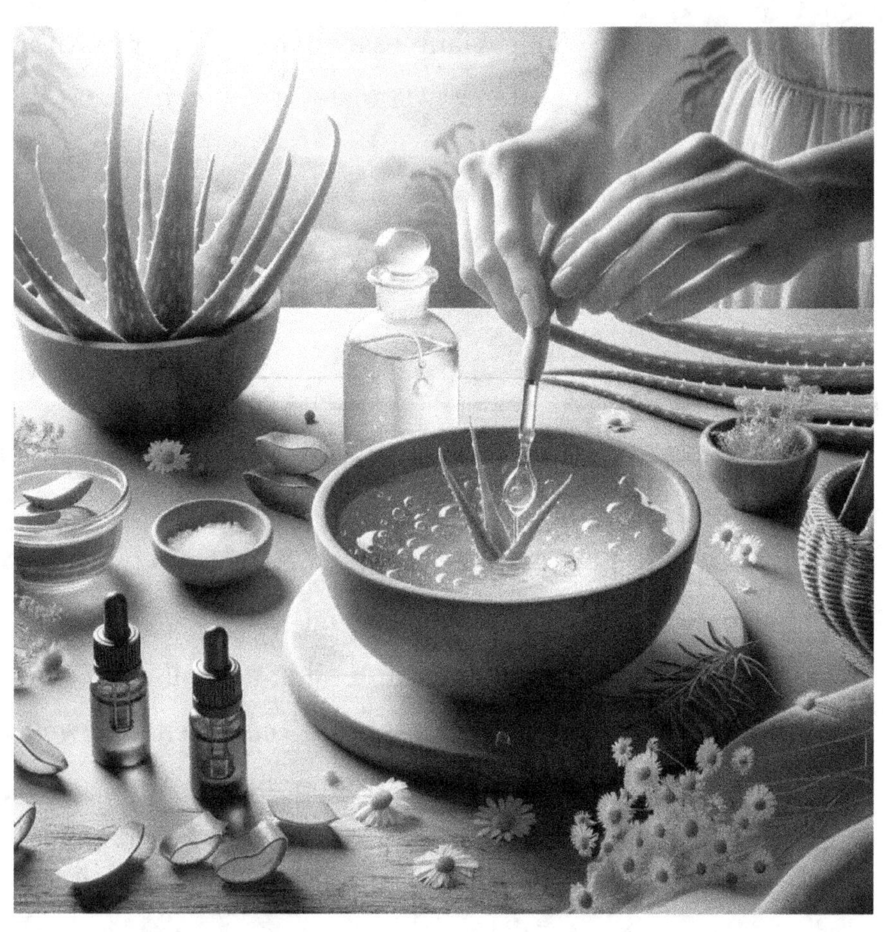

Age-Defying Hyaluronic Acid Serum

P.T.: 20 minutes

Ingr.: 1/4 cup Rosewater, 1 tsp Hyaluronic Acid powder, 10 drops Pomegranate Seed oil, 5 drops Rose essential oil

Process: Dissolve Hyaluronic Acid powder in Rosewater. Stir in Pomegranate Seed oil and Rose essential oil until well combined. Store in a serum bottle. Apply nightly to face and neck for anti-aging benefits.

Brightening Vitamin C Serum

P.T.: 15 minutes

Ingr.: 1/4 cup distilled water, 1 tsp Vitamin C powder (L-Ascorbic Acid), 1 tbsp Glycerin, 10 drops Lemon oil

Process: Dissolve Vitamin C powder in distilled water. Add Glycerin and Lemon essential oil, stirring well. Pour into a dark glass bottle. Use in the morning before moisturizing for a brightening effect.

Calming Green Tea Eye Serum

P.T.: 18 minutes

Ingr.: 1/4 cup brewed Green Tea (cooled), 1 tbsp Almond oil, 5 drops Cucumber Seed oil, 5 drops Green Tea Extract

Process: Mix Green Tea, Almond oil, Cucumber Seed oil, and Green Tea Extract in a bowl. Transfer to a small dropper bottle. Apply gently around the eyes to reduce puffiness and dark circles.

As we conclude our exploration of specialty topical applications, we are left with a deeper appreciation of the natural remedies that can be created right in our homes. This chapter has journeyed through the diverse world of handcrafted salves, lotions, gels, and serums, each offering unique benefits to the skin and senses. These recipes embody the essence of holistic skincare, combining the healing properties of plants with the art of formulation. The insights gained not only equip us with the knowledge to care for our skin naturally but also inspire a deeper connection with the ingredients and their sources. As we move forward, these creations stand as a testament to the beauty and efficacy of natural skincare, encouraging a shift towards more conscious and personalized approaches in our daily routines.

CHAPTER 3: Aromatic Crafts for Wellbeing

In the enchanting world of aromatic crafts, the fusion of fragrance and creativity brings forth an array of delightful products for wellbeing. This chapter serves as a guide into crafting scented candles and wax melts, creating aromatic jewelry and personal adornments, and hand-making soaps and bath products. It's an exploration of how the essence of nature can be captured and infused into everyday items, transforming them into sources of comfort, relaxation, and joy. Each section unveils the step-by-step processes, revealing how simple ingredients, when combined with essential oils, can yield extraordinary results. This journey through aromatic crafts is not just about making products; it's about creating experiences that engage the senses, soothe the soul, and enhance the quality of life.

Scented Candles and Wax Melts

Vanilla Twilight Candle

P.T.: 45 minutes

Ingr.: 1 lb Soy wax, 1 oz Vanilla essential oil, Cotton wick, Candle jar

Process: Melt the soy wax in a double boiler. Once fully melted, remove from heat and stir in the Vanilla essential oil. Center the cotton wick in the candle jar. Pour the wax into the jar, ensuring the wick stays centered. Let it cool and solidify for 24 hours.

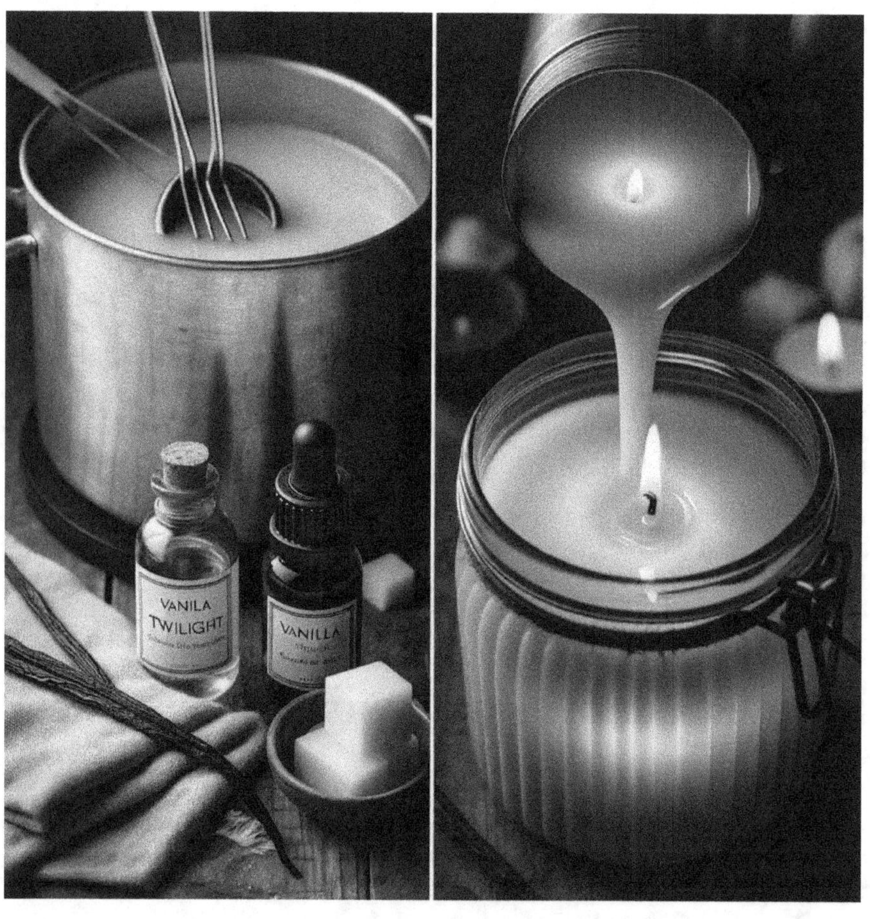

Lavender Dreams Wax Melt

P.T.: 30 minutes

Ingr.: 1/2 lb Beeswax, 1/2 oz Lavender essential oil, Wax melt mold

Process: Gently melt the beeswax in a double boiler. After melting, remove from heat and mix in Lavender essential oil. Pour into wax melt molds. Allow to cool and harden before use.

Eucalyptus Mint Energy Candle

P.T.: 50 minutes

Ingr.: 1 lb Paraffin wax, 0.5 oz Eucalyptus oil, 0.5 oz Peppermint oil, Cotton wick, Glass container

Process: Melt paraffin wax in a double boiler. Once liquid, mix in Eucalyptus and Peppermint oils. Place the wick in a glass container and pour the wax mixture in, keeping the wick straight. Let it set for 24 hours.

Citrus Burst Soy Wax Melts

P.T.: 35 minutes

Ingr.: 1/2 lb Soy wax, 0.25 oz Lemon oil, 0.25 oz Orange oil, Wax melt tray

Process: Melt soy wax over a double boiler. Remove from heat and add Lemon and Orange essential oils. Stir well and pour into a wax melt tray. Let them solidify before use.

P.T.: 45 minutes

Ingr.: 1 lb Coconut wax, 1 oz Rose Geranium essential oil, Wood wick, Decorative candle container

Process: Melt coconut wax in a double boiler. After fully melting, stir in Rose Geranium oil. Place the wood wick in the decorative container, then carefully pour the wax in. Allow to cool and set for a day.

Aromatic Jewelry and Personal Adornments

Lavender Locket Diffuser Necklace

P.T.: 15 minutes

Ingr.: Locket pendant, Small piece of felt, Lavender essential oil

Process: Cut the felt to fit inside the locket. Add a few drops of Lavender essential oil to the felt. Place the scented felt inside the locket. Wear the necklace to enjoy the calming aroma of Lavender throughout the day.

Peppermint Aroma Bracelet

P.T.: 20 minutes

Ingr.: Lava bead bracelet, Peppermint essential oil

Process: Place a few drops of Peppermint essential oil onto the lava beads. Allow the oil to absorb for a few minutes before wearing. The bracelet will release a refreshing Peppermint scent, perfect for energy and focus.

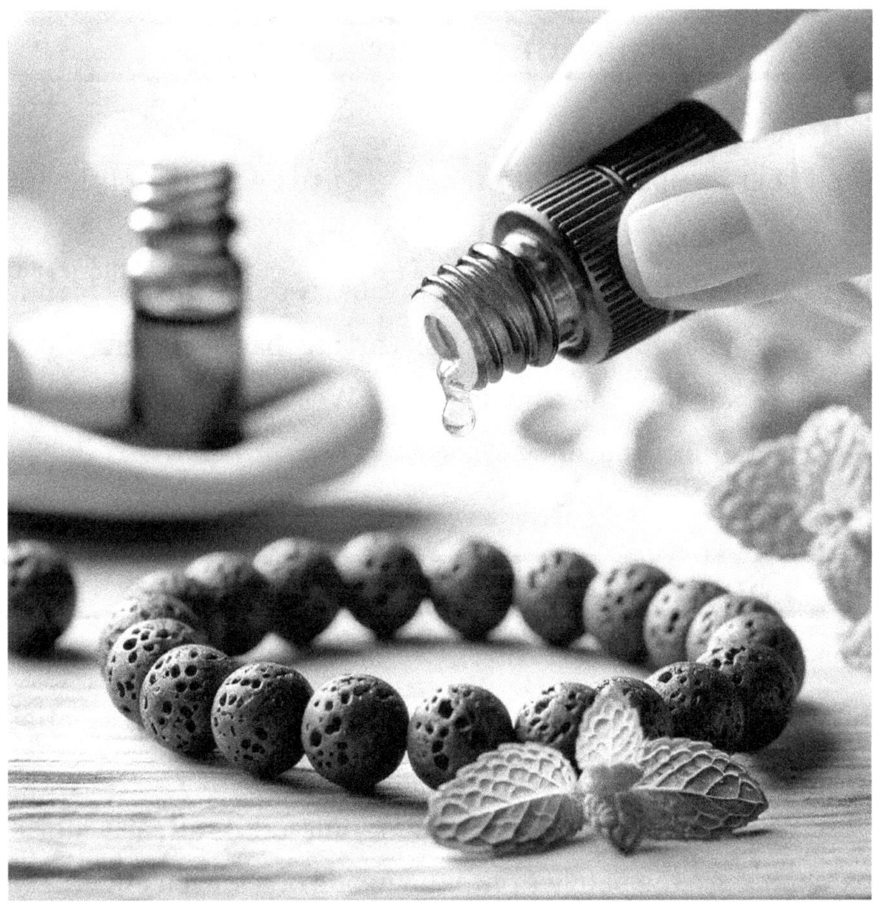

Rose Geranium Aromatic Hairpin

P.T.: 10 minutes

Ingr.: Decorative hairpin, Small cotton pad, Rose Geranium essential oil

Process: Soak the small cotton pad with a few drops of Rose Geranium oil. Attach the pad discreetly to the hairpin. Wear in your hair for a subtle floral fragrance that lasts all day.

Citrus Infused Earring Backs

P.T.: 5 minutes

Ingr.: Earring backs, Cotton swabs, Citrus essential oil blend (Lemon, Orange, Grapefruit)

Process: Soak the tips of cotton swabs in the Citrus oil blend. Trim the soaked tips to fit the earring backs. Insert these scented pads into the earring backs. Wear your earrings for a zesty and uplifting aroma.

Soothing Chamomile Scarf Accents

P.T.: 10 minutes

Ingr.: Small fabric patches, Safety pins, Chamomile essential oil

Process: Add a few drops of Chamomile oil onto each fabric patch. Secure the patches onto the inside of a scarf using safety pins. The scarf will emit a soothing Chamomile fragrance, creating a comforting accessory.

Handmade Soap and Bath Products

Energizing Citrus Shower Gel

P.T.: 30 minutes

Ingr.: 1 cup Unscented liquid Castile soap, 1/4 cup Vegetable glycerin, 15 drops Lemon essential oil, 15 drops Grapefruit essential oil, 10 drops Lime essential oil

Process: In a bowl, mix Castile soap with vegetable glycerin. Stir in Lemon, Grapefruit, and Lime essential oils. Pour the mixture into a pump bottle. Use in the shower for an invigorating and refreshing experience.

Lavender Relaxation Bath Bombs

P.T.: 45 minutes

Ingr.: 1 cup Baking soda, 1/2 cup Citric acid, 1/2 cup Epsom salt, 2 tbsp Almond oil, 20 drops Lavender essential oil, Water in a spray bottle, Bath bomb molds

Process: Mix baking soda, citric acid, and Epsom salt. Add almond oil and Lavender oil, mixing thoroughly. Spritz with water until the mixture holds together when squeezed. Press into molds and let dry for 24 hours before use.

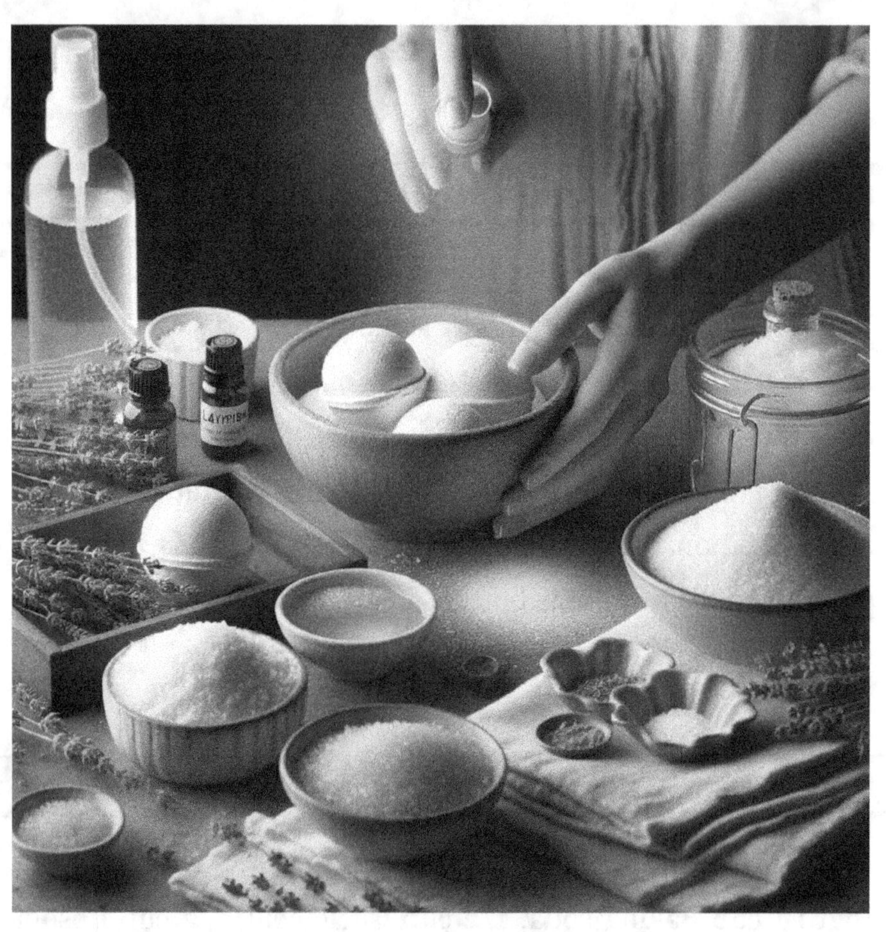

Peppermint Foot Scrub

P.T.: 20 minutes

Ingr.: 1 cup Coarse sea salt, 1/2 cup Coconut oil, 15 drops Peppermint essential oil, 5 drops Tea Tree essential oil

Process: Combine sea salt and coconut oil in a bowl. Stir in Peppermint and Tea Tree oils. Store in a jar. Massage onto feet, focusing on rough areas, then rinse off for smooth, refreshed skin.

Calming Chamomile Soap Bars

P.T.: 1 hour (plus curing time)

Ingr.: 1 lb Soap base (shea butter or glycerin), 1/4 cup Chamomile tea (brewed and cooled), 20 drops Chamomile essential oil, Soap molds

Process: Melt the soap base in a double boiler. Stir in cooled Chamomile tea and Chamomile oil. Pour into molds and let set until hardened. Allow the bars to cure in a dry area for a few weeks before use.

Rose and Honey Bubble Bath

P.T.: 25 minutes

Ingr.: 1 cup Liquid Castile soap, 1/3 cup Raw honey, 1/4 cup Rosewater, 15 drops Rose essential oil

Process: Gently warm honey to make it runny, but not hot. In a bowl, mix liquid Castile soap, rosewater, and warm honey. Stir in Rose essential oil. Pour into a bottle. Add to running bath water for a luxurious, bubbly soak.

As we conclude our journey through the art of aromatic crafting, we are left with a treasure trove of knowledge and inspiration. This chapter has unveiled the secrets of creating fragrant masterpieces that enrich our lives and environments. From the soothing glow of handmade candles to the personal touch of scented jewelry, and the luxury of natural bath products, each craft is a testament to the beauty and versatility of essential oils. These creations are more than just hobbies; they are pathways to wellness, offering therapeutic benefits that soothe, rejuvenate, and uplift. Moving forward, the skills and recipes gleaned from this chapter empower us to incorporate the essence of aromatherapy into our daily routines, enhancing our wellbeing and bringing a touch of handmade elegance to our world.

CHAPTER 4: Aromatherapy for Special Populations

Embarking on a journey through the realm of aromatherapy for special populations, this chapter presents a nuanced understanding of how essential oils can be tailored to meet the unique needs of diverse groups. It explores the delicate art of creating blends for children and the elderly, addressing their specific health and emotional requirements with gentleness and care. The chapter then transitions to the dynamic world of athletes, highlighting how aromatherapy can enhance physical performance and recovery. Finally, it delves into the supportive role of essential oils in mental health, offering natural ways to alleviate stress, anxiety, and other psychological challenges. This exploration is a testament to the versatility and adaptability of aromatherapy, demonstrating its potential to provide comfort and healing across various stages of life and conditions.

Blends for Children and the Elderly

Gentle Dreams Blend for Children

P.T.: 10 minutes

Ingr.: 2 tbsp Fractionated Coconut oil, 3 drops Lavender oil, 2 drops Roman Chamomile oil, 1 drop Frankincense oil

Process: Mix the essential oils into the Fractionated Coconut oil in a small bottle. Gently shake to blend. Apply a small amount to the child's wrists or feet before bedtime for a soothing, restful sleep.

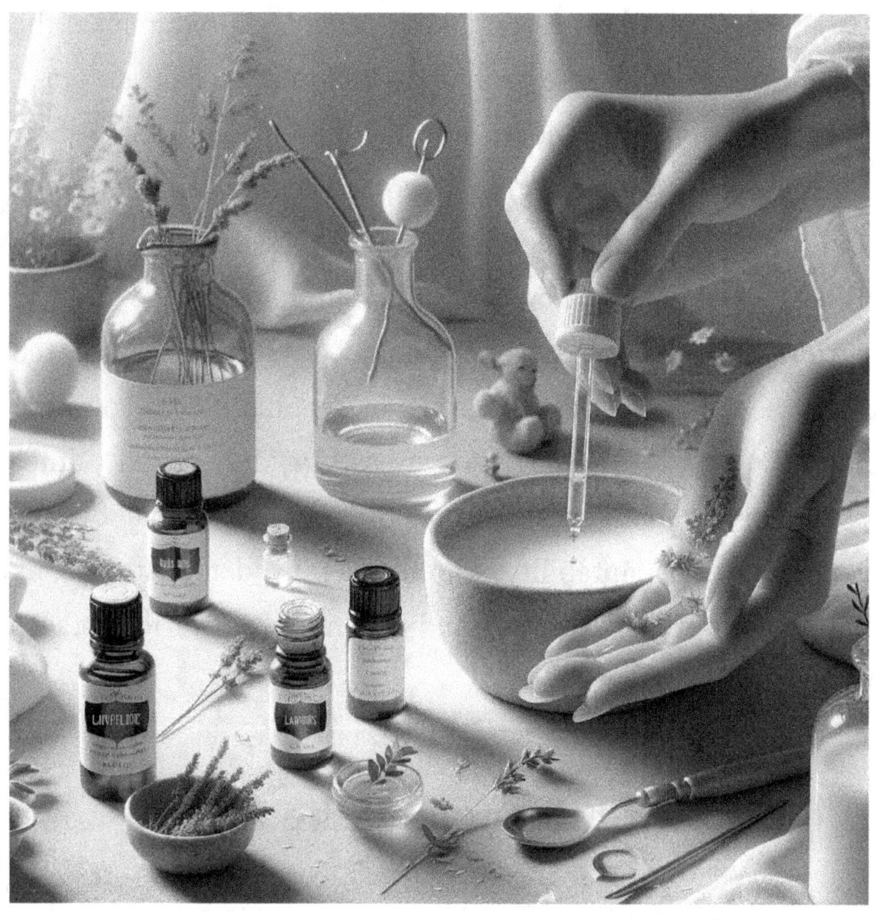

Memory Boost Blend for the Elderly

P.T.: 12 minutes

Ingr.: 2 tbsp Jojoba oil, 3 drops Rosemary oil, 2 drops Peppermint oil, 2 drops Lemon oil

Process: Blend the essential oils with Jojoba oil in a dark glass bottle. Shake well. Use by applying to the temples and back of the neck to aid memory and concentration.

Calming Blend for Children

P.T.: 8 minutes

Ingr.: 2 tbsp Almond oil, 3 drops Mandarin oil, 2 drops Cedarwood oil, 1 drop Neroli oil

Process: Combine all oils in a small bottle and shake to mix. Apply to the child's chest or back, or use in a diffuser at a low setting to calm and comfort.

Joint Relief Blend for the Elderly

P.T.: 15 minutes

Ingr.: 3 tbsp Olive oil, 4 drops Ginger oil, 3 drops Eucalyptus oil, 2 drops Black Pepper oil

Process: Mix the essential oils with Olive oil in a bottle. Shake to blend thoroughly. Massage gently into joints to help alleviate discomfort and improve mobility.

Soothing Skin Blend for Elderly Skin

P.T.: 10 minutes

Ingr.: 2 tbsp Avocado oil, 3 drops Helichrysum oil, 2 drops Lavender oil, 1 drop Tea Tree oil

Process: Combine the oils in a small container. Stir well. Apply to areas of dry or irritated skin to soothe and moisturize.

Aromatherapy for Athletes

Muscle Recovery Blend

P.T.: 10 minutes

Ingr.: 3 tbsp Grapeseed oil, 5 drops Marjoram oil, 5 drops Rosemary oil, 4 drops Lavender oil

Process: Combine all the oils in a bottle. Shake well to blend. Apply to muscles post-workout with a gentle massage to aid in recovery and reduce soreness.

Energy Boost Inhaler

P.T.: 5 minutes

Ingr.: Aromatherapy inhaler, 5 drops Peppermint oil, 5 drops Lemon oil, 3 drops Eucalyptus oil

Process: Add the essential oils to the cotton wick of the inhaler. Assemble the inhaler. Use before or during workouts for an instant energy boost.

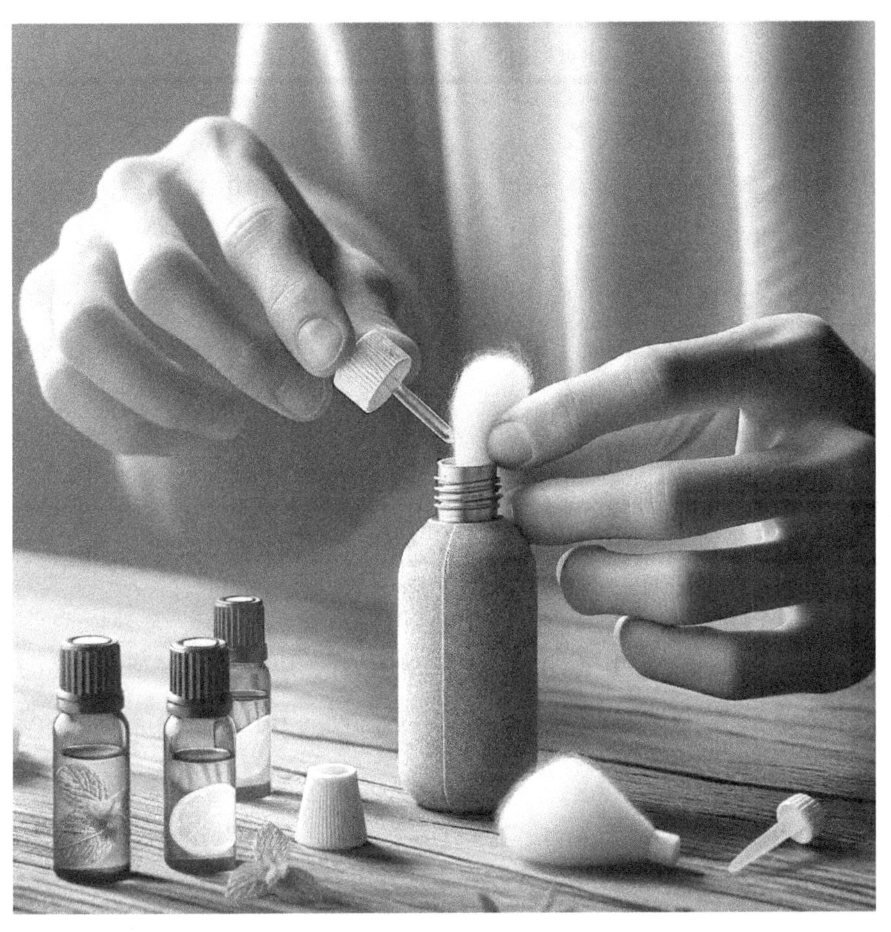

Focus and Stamina Roller Blend

P.T.: 7 minutes

Ingr.: 10ml Roller bottle, 2 tbsp Fractionated Coconut oil, 4 drops Frankincense oil, 4 drops Wild Orange oil, 3 drops Peppermint oil

Process: Fill the roller bottle with Fractionated Coconut oil. Add the essential oils. Shake well. Roll onto pulse points before athletic activities to enhance focus and stamina.

Cooling Foot Soak

P.T.: 10 minutes

Ingr.: 1/2 cup Epsom salt, 5 drops Peppermint oil, 5 drops Lavender oil, 3 drops Tea Tree oil

Process: Mix Epsom salt with the essential oils. Dissolve in warm water in a foot bath. Soak feet post-exercise to refresh and cool tired feet.

Post-Workout Shower Gel

P.T.: 15 minutes

Ingr.: 1 cup Unscented liquid Castile soap, 1/4 cup Aloe Vera gel, 10 drops Ginger oil, 10 drops Cypress oil, 5 drops Juniper Berry oil

Process: Mix Castile soap with Aloe Vera gel. Stir in the essential oils. Store in a squeeze bottle. Use in the shower post-exercise to invigorate and support muscle relaxation.

Supporting Mental Health with Aromatherapy

The intricate realm of mental health, a vital component of our overall well-being, finds a nurturing ally in aromatherapy. This ancient practice transcends its roots of simply providing pleasant scents; it becomes a holistic tool that taps into the very essence of nature to heal and soothe the mind. Delving into the world of essential oils reveals their capacity to alleviate stress, anxiety, depression, and other mental health challenges, offering a natural adjunct to traditional therapies.

Central to the effectiveness of aromatherapy in mental health is the understanding that our sense of smell is directly linked to the limbic system of the brain, which governs emotions and memories. This direct pathway enables essential oils to influence our mental state subtly yet significantly. The right aromatic blend can provide comfort and relief, offering a sense of tranquility in the midst of mental turmoil.

Consider the calming properties of Lavender (Lavandula angustifolia). In today's fast-paced world, where stress and anxiety are common, Lavender stands as a beacon of calmness. Its gentle aroma acts as a soothing embrace, quieting the mind and easing nervous tension. Moments of overwhelm are softened by the inhalation of this fragrance, providing a peaceful respite.

Bergamot (Citrus bergamia), with its uplifting qualities, brings light to darker days marked by depression or melancholy. Its citrusy scent acts as a natural antidepressant, promoting joy and renewing energy. The presence of Bergamot can be akin to a sunbeam, breaking through the clouds of despair, uplifting the spirit.

Peppermint (Mentha piperita) is celebrated for enhancing mental clarity and focus. Amidst a world teeming with distractions, maintaining sharp concentration can be challenging. Peppermint, with its revitalizing aroma, acts as a mental stimulant, clearing foggy thoughts, sharpening focus, and improving cognitive performance. It is particularly valuable for those struggling with attention deficits.

Roman Chamomile (Anthemis nobilis) offers a natural solution to insomnia, a common companion of mental health issues. Its gentle, apple-like fragrance lulls the restless mind, promoting a peaceful and restorative sleep. In the quiet of the night, Roman Chamomile becomes a gentle lullaby, leading the way to a tranquil rest.

Crafting blends for mental health is an art that involves understanding each individual's emotional and psychological landscape. It's about selecting oils that resonate with the person's unique needs, creating a harmonious blend that speaks to their soul. Whether it's a concoction to elevate mood, soothe the mind, boost concentration, or encourage sleep, each blend is a testament to the power of natural fragrances in supporting mental wellness.

Aromatherapy, in the context of mental health, is a journey of exploration and healing. It opens a path where the fragrances of nature become more than just scents; they transform into tools for healing, guiding us toward mental equilibrium and peace. This exploration into essential oils and mental health care invites us to embrace the healing powers of nature, providing a complementary approach to traditional mental health therapies.

Conclusion

As we reach the end of our journey through 'The Essential Oils and Remedies Bible for Everyday Use,' it's important to step back and reflect on the profound insights and wisdom we've gleaned. This book has not just been a guide; it's been a gateway into a world where nature's essence brings healing, comfort, and rejuvenation to our daily lives. The journey through these pages has illuminated the myriad ways in which essential oils can enrich our existence, touching every aspect of our being – physical, emotional, and spiritual.

From the very first chapter, where we delved into the history and renaissance of aromatherapy, we embarked on a path of discovery, unearthing the ancient roots and modern advancements of this timeless practice. We learned how the distillation and extraction methods bring out the pure essence of nature's bounty, providing us with the very soul of plants in the form of essential oils. Understanding the purity and quality of these oils opened our eyes to their true potential and value.

The exploration of aromatic remedies and therapeutic applications brought to light the profound healing capabilities of essential oils. We saw how they can be integrated into various aspects of daily life, offering natural alternatives for holistic well-being. Whether it was through the soothing touch of a massage oil or the invigorating scent of a diffuser blend, we learned how essential oils could become our allies in navigating the complexities of modern life.

The journey through this book also took us into the intimate spaces of our homes, where we learned to craft personal care potions and holistic home care solutions. From nourishing skin care recipes to eco-friendly cleaning solutions, we discovered the versatility of essential oils in enhancing the health and harmony of our living environments.

One of the most compelling revelations of this book was the way essential oils bridge the gap between the ancient and the modern. We delved into the world of advanced aromatherapy, exploring the chemical constituents and synergy of essential oils. We unraveled the science behind the scents, demystifying how these aromatic compounds interact with our bodies and minds to elicit profound therapeutic effects.

Building an aromatherapy brand and navigating the business landscape of essential oils highlighted the importance of ethical sourcing, sustainability, and compliance. This knowledge is crucial not only for entrepreneurs but also for consumers, fostering a more informed and conscious approach to choosing and using essential oils.

This book also opened our eyes to the specific needs of different populations, underscoring the adaptability and sensitivity of aromatherapy practices. From blends tailored for children and the elderly to those designed for athletes and individuals seeking mental health support, we learned how essential oils could be customized to meet diverse needs.

As we close this chapter of our aromatic exploration, it's clear that the journey doesn't end here. The world of essential oils is vast and ever-evolving, with each day bringing new research, insights, and applications. The knowledge we've acquired from this book lays a foundation, but the learning continues as we experiment, experience, and grow in our understanding and application of essential oils.

It's important to remember that our journey with essential oils is deeply personal and unique. What works for one may not work for another, and part of the beauty of aromatherapy lies in this individual exploration and discovery. We encourage you to keep experimenting with different oils and blends, listening to your body and mind, and finding what resonates best with you.

As we conclude, let us carry forward the spirit of respect and reverence for nature that has been a constant theme in this book. Let us continue to harness the gifts of the earth responsibly and sustainably, honoring the plants and the ancient wisdom that has been passed down through generations. In doing so, we not only enrich our own lives but also contribute to the well-being of our planet and future generations.

'The Essential Oils and Remedies Bible for Everyday Use' is more than a book; it's a companion on your journey toward natural wellness. May the scents of the earth bring you peace, health, and joy as you continue to explore the wonderful world of aromatherapy.